T0326316

Curbside Consultation

of the Liver

49 Clinical Questions

CURBSIDE CONSULTATION IN GASTROENTEROLOGY
SERIES

SERIES EDITOR, FRANCIS A. FARRAYE, MD, MSC, FACP, FACG

Curbside Consultation
of the Liver

49 Clinical Questions

EDITED BY

MITCHELL L. SHIFFMAN, MD
PROFESSOR OF MEDICINE
CHIEF, HEPATOLOGY SECTION
MEDICAL DIRECTOR, LIVER TRANSPLANTATION PROGRAM
VIRGINIA COMMONWEALTH UNIVERSITY MEDICAL CENTER
RICHMOND, VIRGINIA

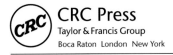

CRC Press
Taylor & Francis Group
Boca Raton London New York

CRC Press is an imprint of the
Taylor & Francis Group, an **informa** business

First published 2008 by SLACK Incorporated

Published 2024 by CRC Press
2385 NW Executive Center Drive, Suite 320, Boca Raton FL 33431

and by CRC Press
4 Park Square, Milton Park, Abingdon, Oxon, OX14 4RN

CRC Press is an imprint of Taylor & Francis Group, LLC

© 2008 Taylor & Francis Group, LLC

Library of Congress Cataloging-in-Publication Data

Curbside consultation of the liver : 49 clinical questions / edited by Mitchell L. Shiffman.
    p. ; cm.
  Includes bibliographical references and index.
  ISBN 9781556428159 (softcover : alk. paper) 1. Liver--Diseases--Handbooks, manuals, etc. I. Shiffman, Mitchell L.
  [DNLM: 1. Liver Diseases. WI 700 C975 2008]
  RC846.C87 2008
  616.3′62--dc22
                          2008005781

ISBN: 9781556428159 (pbk)
ISBN: 9781003523758 (ebk)

DOI: 10.1201/9781003523758

Dedication

This book is dedicated to all the gastroenterologists and primary care providers throughout Virginia who regularly refer and entrust the care of their patients to our Hepatology group at the Virginia Commonwealth University Medical Center.

Contents

SECTION III: LIVER DISEASE IN PATIENTS WITH HIV INFECTION

SECTION IV: GENETIC DISORDERS THAT CAUSE CHRONIC LIVER DISEASE

SECTION VII: CIRRHOSIS

SECTION VIII: LIVER TRANSPLANTATION

Acknowledgments

I would like to thank A. Scott Mills, MD, our long time Pathology colleague and collaborator, for supplying the pictures utilized for the cover of this book.

About the Editor

Mitchell L. Shiffman, MD received his MD degree from the State University of New York, Upstate Medical Center in Syracuse, NY. He then completed internship and residency training in Internal Medicine at the Medical College of Virginia (now the Virginia Commonwealth University Medical Center) in Richmond, VA. He remained at this institution for fellowship training in Gastroenterology and Hepatology, which included two years of research training funded by a National Institutes of Health training grant. After completing his training, Dr. Shiffman joined the faculty of the Virginia Commonwealth University as an Assistant Professor of Medicine and has remained at this institution throughout his academic career. He is currently a Professor of Medicine, and has been the Chief of the Hepatology Section and Medical Director of the Liver Transplant Program at the VCU Medical Center for over a decade.

Dr. Shiffman has authored or coauthored over 200 original articles, editorials, reviews, and/or book chapters. His clinical research has focused on improving our understanding and developing better treatments for viral hepatitis B and C. He is a member of the Board of Trustees of the American College of Gastroenterology, and has served on numerous NIH grant review committees and is a member of the Editorial Boards of *Liver Transplantation* and *Liver International*.

Contributing Authors

Paul Arnold, MD
Fellow in Gastroenterology
Division of Gastroenterology, Hepatology,
  and Nutrition
Virginia Commonwealth University
  School of Medicine
Richmond, VA

Ramesh Ashwath, MD
Fellow in Gastroenterology
Division of Gastroenterology, Hepatology,
  and Nutrition
Virginia Commonwealth University
  School of Medicine
Richmond, VA

Lawrence Chang, MD
Attending Physician
Central Dupage Hospital
Winfield, IL

Opang Cheung, MD
Fellow in Gastroenterology
Division of Gastroenterology, Hepatology,
  and Nutrition
Virginia Commonwealth University
  School of Medicine
Richmond, VA

Jayanta Choudhury, MD
Fellow in Gastroenterology
Division of Gastroenterology, Hepatology,
  and Nutrition
Virginia Commonwealth University
  School of Medicine
Richmond, VA

Kevin M. Comar, MD
Fellow in Gastroenterology
Division of Gastroenterology, Hepatology,
  and Nutrition
Virginia Commonwealth University
  School of Medicine
Richmond, VA

Peter Dienhart, MD
Fellow in Gastroenterology
Division of Gastroenterology, Hepatology,
  and Nutrition
Virginia Commonwealth University
  School of Medicine
Richmond, VA

Michael Fuchs, MD, PhD, FEBG
Associate Professor of Medicine
Virginia Commonwealth University
  Medical Center
Richmond, VA

Leslie M. Gallagher, MS, ANP
Division of Gastroenterology
McGuire Veterans Administration Medical
  Center
Richmond, VA

HoChong S. Gilles, MS, FNP
Division of Gastroenterology
McGuire Veterans Administration Medical
  Center
Richmond, VA

Adil Habib, MD
Gastroenterology/Hepatology Section
Medical Service (III G)
Overton Brooks VA Medical Center
Shreveport, LA

Douglas M. Heuman, MD
Professor of Medicine
Virginia Commonwealth University
Chief, Hepatology
McGuire Veterans Administration Medical
  Center
Richmond, VA

Wei Hou, MD
Fellow in Gastroenterology
Division of Gastroenterology, Hepatology,
  and Nutrition
Virginia Commonwealth University
  School of Medicine
Richmond, VA

Velimir A. Luketic, MD
Professor of Medicine
Division of Gastroenterology, Hepatology,
  and Nutrition
Virginia Commonwealth University
  Medical Center
Richmond, VA

Anastasios A. Mihas, MD, FACT, FACG
Professor of Medicine
Virginia Commonwealth University
McGuire Veterans Administration Medical
  Center
Richmond, VA

Andres Mogollon, MD
Fellow in Gastroenterology
Division of Gastroenterology, Hepatology,
  and Nutrition
Virginia Commonwealth University
  School of Medicine
Richmond, VA

Puneet Puri, MD
Fellow in Gastroenterology
Division of Gastroenterology, Hepatology,
  and Nutrition
Virginia Commonwealth University
  School of Medicine
Richmond, VA

Seela Ramesh, MD
Fellow in Gastroenterology
Division of Gastroenterology, Hepatology,
  and Nutrition
Virginia Commonwealth University
  School of Medicine
Richmond, VA

B. Marie Reid, MD
Fellow in Gastroenterology
Division of Gastroenterology, Hepatology,
  and Nutrition
Virginia Commonwealth University
  School of Medicine
Richmond, VA

Arun J. Sanyal, MD
Professor of Medicine
Chief, Department of Gastroenterology
  and Hepatology
Virginia Commonwealth University
  Medical Center
Richmond, VA

Amreita Sethi, MD
Fellow in Gastroenterology
Division of Gastroenterology, Hepatology,
  and Nutrition
Virginia Commonwealth University
  School of Medicine
Richmond, VA

Richard K. Sterling, MD, FACP, FACG
Professor of Medicine and Infectious
  Diseases
Virginia Commonwealth University
  Medical Center
Richmond, VA

R. Todd Stravitz, MD
Associate Professor of Medicine
Virginia Commonwealth University
  Medical Center
Richmond, VA

Nogib Toubia, MD
Fellow in Gastroenterology
Division of Gastroenterology, Hepatology,
  and Nutrition
Virginia Commonwealth University
  School of Medicine
Richmond, VA

Preface

When I was first approached by SLACK Incorporated about developing and editing a textbook in Hepatology, I really did not think there was a need for yet another text in this field. After all, the field is very narrow and there were already many excellent Hepatology texts in print. For the most part, these books are large, deal with virtually every aspect of liver disease, are heavily referenced and contain detailed and excellent explanations of disease pathophysiology. I have many of these texts on the bookshelf behind my desk. Unfortunately, many busy gastroenterologists often find it difficult and frustrating to find concise answers to many basic clinical questions in these reference texts.

Curbside Consultation of the Liver: 49 Clinical Questions represents a unique format and is quite different than any of these reference Hepatology texts. Each chapter title is a simple commonly asked question related to a specific aspect of liver disease. All of these questions have been posed to me by either gastroenterologists and/or primary care providers who have regularly referred patients to our Hepatology group practice at the Virginia Commonwealth University Medical Center over the past several years. The chapter itself, provides a definitive answer to this question with a relatively brief and focused explanation in a format that is easy to read and only lightly referenced. All of these explanations contain the opinions of the authors and reflect the manner in which our Hepatology group practices and would approach this issue in our own patients.

As the name of our text implies, *Curbside Consultation of the Liver: 49 Clinical Questions* contains 49 clinical questions divided into 8 Sections; Hepatitis C Virus, Hepatitis B Virus, Liver Disease in Patients with HIV Infection, Genetic Disorders which Cause Chronic Liver Disease, Fatty Liver Disease, Cholestatic Liver Diseases, Cirrhosis, and Liver Transplantation. Each of these chapters has been authored by a member of our own Hepatology faculty; and each the fellows in our Gastroenterology and Hepatology fellowship program contributed as co-authors to many of these chapters. This represents yet another unique aspect of this book—it is entirely written and edited by the physicians of a single academic practice.

It was very difficult selecting only 49 questions to address in this text. The book could have easily been contained 58, or even 62, clinical questions. However, I am confident that we have identified and provided answers to many of the questions that arise when you encounter and treat patients with chronic liver disease in your practice; and that you will find this text to be a useful addition to your reference collection. Finally, I encourage you to provide feedback regarding the usefulness of this text through the publisher. I also welcome your suggestions regarding common questions that I failed to include or difficult questions that you have been unable to find an answer to in the literature. I am hopeful that these questions will provide to foundation for the next 49 clinical questions.

Mitchell L. Shiffman, MD

SECTION I

VIRAL HEPATITIS C

WHAT IS THE LIKELIHOOD THAT MY PATIENT WITH CHRONIC HEPATITIS C WILL DEVELOP CIRRHOSIS, HEPATOCELLULAR CARCINOMA, AND/OR HEPATIC DECOMPENSATION?

Seela Ramesh, MD
Mitchell L. Shiffman, MD

Approximately 4 million persons within the United States are infected with the hepatitis C virus (HCV). Chronic HCV is the most common cause of cirrhosis and hepatocellular carcinoma (HCC), and over 40% of all patients who undergo liver transplantation in the United States, Europe, Canada, Australia, and many countries have chronic HCV infection.[1] Despite this, the natural history of chronic HCV has a wide spectrum. Only 4% of persons with chronic HCV develop end-stage liver disease and/or HCC and need to consider liver transplantation as a therapeutic option (Figure 1-1). To some this may not sound like a major health problem. However, with 4 million persons infected, it is anticipated that 160,000 persons will develop end-stage disease and need to consider liver transplantation within the next 1 to 2 decades. Unfortunately, only about 5000 to 6000 liver transplants are performed in the United States annually, and roughly half of these are in patients without chronic HCV. It would therefore require 50 to 65 years for all those patients with end-stage liver disease from chronic HCV to receive a liver transplant. Clearly, this is an impossible task and many of these patients will not survive the pretransplant waiting period.

When patients first find out they have chronic HCV, the vast majority are afraid that they already have cirrhosis, will develop cirrhosis or HCC, require a liver transplant, and/or die within the next 1 to 2 years. Educating patients regarding the natural history of chronic HCV is one of the most important things that a physician can do for a

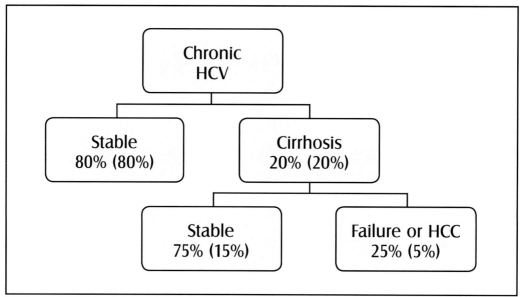

Figure 1-1. The natural history of patients following chronic HCV. Numbers in parentheses reflect the percentage of the total group of persons with chronic HCV infection.

patient with recently diagnosed chronic HCV. As already noted above, the vast majority of patients with chronic HCV will not develop end-stage liver disease. It is therefore imperative that the physician be able to recognize which patients with chronic HCV are at increased risk to develop cirrhosis and to counsel all patients accordingly.

The natural history of chronic HCV and cirrhosis is now well established. Our understanding of this is based upon prospective long-term natural history studies initiated in the 1970s prior to the development of interferon therapy and cross-sectional studies of patients with chronic HCV being evaluated for HCV treatment. As depicted in Figure 1-2, patients with chronic HCV can be divided into one of three groups: (1) patients who will never develop any fibrosis; (2) patients with rapid fibrosis progression who develop cirrhosis within 20 to 30 years after being exposed to HCV; and (3) patients with slow fibrosis progression who would eventually develop cirrhosis but at much slower rates, which would require 30 years or more following exposure. Many persons in this later category may endure 50 to 60 years of chronic HCV infection before they develop cirrhosis. Chronic HCV may therefore not cause morbidity or contribute to mortality in these patients until they reach the seventh or eighth decades of life. During this entire time the great majority of patients with chronic HCV infection are asymptomatic.

The use of liver biopsy and examination of liver histology has traditionally been utilized to assess the risk of developing cirrhosis. The role of liver biopsy in the assessment of patients with chronic HCV is discussed in Question 3. The largest prospective study to evaluate fibrosis progression was initiated in the 1970s prior to the identification of HCV.[2] This study enrolled patients with non-A, non-B hepatitis, over 95% of whom tested positive for HCV when this assay became available in the early 1990s. After an initial liver biopsy, these patients were followed prospectively for 20 years. Repeat liver biopsy was performed after 10 and 20 years or when these patients were thought to have developed cirrhosis based upon clinical grounds. All patients with bridging fibrosis on the initial

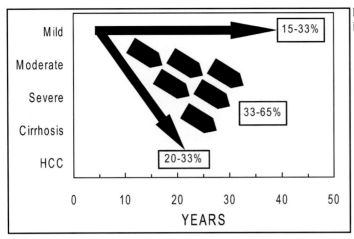

Figure 1-2. Fibrosis progression in patients with chronic HCV.

liver biopsy developed cirrhosis within 5 to 10 years. All patients with portal fibrosis also developed cirrhosis, but this required 10 to 20 years. In contrast, less than 25% of patients with no fibrosis on the initial biopsy developed cirrhosis within 20 years. It is therefore apparent that patients with any degree of fibrosis will progress and eventually develop cirrhosis. Although this may take nearly 2 decades in some patients, it remains unclear how to identify those patients who will progress. This is why it is recommended that patients with any degree of fibrosis on liver biopsy be offered treatment with peginterferon and ribavirin. Waiting until patients "declare themselves" by developing more fibrosis is not recommended since sustained virologic response following treatment with peginterferon and ribavirin has been shown to be inversely related to the degree of fibrosis on liver biopsy. In contrast, the vast majority of patients with no fibrosis on liver biopsy will not develop cirrhosis over the next 2 decades or longer. The majority of these patients have normal liver transaminases (see Question 2).

Population-based studies have identified several risk factors associated with the development of cirrhosis.[3] These include acquiring HCV at a later age, obesity, human immunodeficiency virus (HIV) coinfection, and having a concomitant liver disease such as HBV coinfection, hemochromatosis, nonalcoholic steatohepatitis, or being homozygous or heterozygous for alpha-1-antitrypsin deficiency. Regular alcohol use is frequently listed as a factor that accelerates the progression of chronic HCV to cirrhosis and increases the risk of developing HCC. While this is likely to be correct for persons who consume more than 6 alcoholic beverages per day, it remains unclear and controversial whether smaller amounts of alcohol, 1 drink per day or less, impact the natural history of chronic HCV.[4]

A genetic test has recently been developed that may allow physicians to identify those patients with chronic HCV who will develop fibrosis progression.[5] This genetic test is performed on whole blood and assesses for certain single nucleotide polymorphisms (SNPs) in 7 genes, some of which are related to hepatic inflammation and fibrosis. The pattern of SNPs in these 7 genes is then converted into a numerical score that correlates with the risk of developing advanced fibrosis and cirrhosis. The Cirrhosis Risk Score (CRS) will soon be commercially available and can be utilized to identify patients who will progress to cirrhosis. Patients with a high CRS need not undergo a liver biopsy and can simply be considered for HCV treatment.

The natural history of cirrhosis in patients with chronic HCV has been evaluated in prospective clinical trials conducted over several decades prior to the availability of interferon.[6] In one of these studies, 380 patients with a Child-Pugh-Turcotte (CPT) score of 6 or less and without any prior complications of cirrhosis were followed for up to 10 years. Overall, over 80% of these patients were alive after 10 years of follow-up. In contrast, patients who had either a decline in the CTP score or developed complications of cirrhosis had a marked decline in survival; approximately 50% of patients with decompensated cirrhosis died within 5 years and only 30% remained alive after 10 years. Thus, patients should be referred to a liver transplant program as soon as they develop a CPT score of 7 or greater and/or if a complication of cirrhosis such as variceal hemorrhage, ascites, hepatic encephalopathy, or HCC develops. Approximately 3% to 5% of patients with stable cirrhosis will develop complications of cirrhosis and another 1% to 3% will develop HCC on an annual basis. Thus, after 5 years of following a group of patients with stable cirrhosis, 20% would be expected to have developed hepatic decompensation and 10% to have developed HCC. Thus, patients with chronic HCV and cirrhosis need to be monitored at periodic intervals for evidence of hepatic decompensation and to screen for HCC. In our own practice we see these patients every 3 to 6 months to assess liver function and to screen for HCC. The latter is discussed in Question 39.

In summary, the vast majority of patients with chronic HCV develop progressive fibrosis and a significant proportion will develop cirrhosis. Assessing the degree of fibrosis by performing a liver biopsy is very helpful in assessing this risk and counseling patients. The cirrhosis risk score may prove to be very useful in identifying patients with significant risk for developing cirrhosis and reduce the need for liver biopsy. Approximately 3% to 5% of HCV patients with stable cirrhosis are at risk to develop hepatic decompensation per year; another 1% to 3% will develop HCC. As a result, monitoring and screening patients with HCV and cirrhosis on a regular basis are imperative. Since patients with any degree of fibrosis are at risk to progress, all such patients should be considered candidates for treatment with peginterferon and ribavirin.

References

1. Kim WR. The burden of hepatitis C in the United States. *Hepatology*. 2002;36(5 Suppl 1):S30-S34.
2. Yano M, Kumada H, Kage M, et al. The long term pathological evolution of chronic hepatitis C. *Hepatology*. 1996;23:1334-1340.
3. Poynard T, Bedossa P, Opolon P. Natural history of liver fibrosis progression in patients with chronic hepatitis C. *Lancet*. 1997;349:825-832.
4. Monto A, Patel K, Bostrom A, et al. Risks of a range of alcohol intake on hepatitis C–related fibrosis. *Hepatology*. 2004;39:826-834.
5. Huang H, Shiffman ML, Friedman S, et al. A 7 gene signature identifies the risk of developing cirrhosis in patients with chronic hepatitis C. *Hepatology*. 2007;46:297-306
6. Fattovich G, Giustina G, Degos F, et al. Morbidity and mortality in compensated and cirrhosis type C: a retrospective follow-up study of 384 patients. *Gastroenterology*. 1997;112:463-472.

QUESTION

2

HOW SHOULD A PATIENT WHO TESTS POSITIVE FOR CHRONIC HEPATITIS C BUT HAS PERSISTENTLY NORMAL SERUM AMINOTRANSAMINASES BE EVALUATED?

Ramesh Ashwath, MD
Mitchell L. Shiffman, MD

Approximately 20% to 33% of patients with chronic hepatitis C virus (HCV) infection have persistently normal aminotransferase activity (PNAT). Historically, these patients were felt to have "milder" HCV and thought to be "less likely" to develop fibrosis progression and cirrhosis compared to patients with elevated aminotransferases (AT) activity. In addition, scattered brief reports demonstrated that some patients with PNAT developed elevations in serum AT activity during treatment. As a result of these observations, the first National Institute Health Consensus Conference on HCV in 1997 recommended that patients with PNAT be monitored but not treated. During the past decade, numerous studies have closely evaluated the natural history of HCV in patients with PNAT and controlled clinical treatment trials have evaluated the impact of peginterferon and ribavirin in these patients.

What Is the Natural History of a PNAT in Patients With Chronic HCV?

Several studies have investigated the natural history of patients with chronic HCV and PNAT. These patients are more commonly female, but there appears to be no relationship to genotype or the serum level of HCV RNA.[1] When compared to patients with elevated serum AT, patients with PNAT tend to have milder liver injury on liver biopsy. However, approximately 33% to 75% of patients with PNAT have variable degrees of fibrosis and anywhere from 2% to 5% have cirrhosis[2] (Figure 2-1). Patients with PNAT

Figure 2-1. Histologic spectrum of patients with chronic HCV and PNAT (Adapted from Puoti C, Castellacci R, Montagnese F, et al. Histological and virological features and follow-up of hepatitis C virus carriers with normal aminotransferase levels: the Italian prospective study of the asymptomatic C carriers (ISACC). *J Hepatol.* 2002;37:117-123).

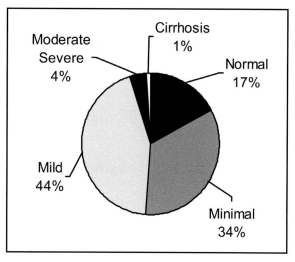

may also develop fibrosis progression, although the rate of progression does appear to be somewhat slower than in patients with elevated AT. A prospective study demonstrated that patients with elevated AT all developed fibrosis progression over 10 to 15 years. In contrast, fibrosis progression was observed in only 30% of patients with PNAT.[3] Those patients with PNAT who did not develop fibrosis progression had no fibrosis on the initial liver biopsy.

It is well known that serum AT may fluctuate widely in patients with chronic HCV. The same appears to be true of HCV patients with a PNAT. In a study of 800 patients with HCV documented to have PNAT over 1 year, 24% of these patients had a flare in serum AT to values above the upper limit of normal within the next 3 years.[4] Some of these flares represented only a single elevation in AT, which returned to the normal range the next time this was evaluated. However, some flares lasted several months before returning to the normal range or the serum AT remained persistently elevated. These flares were not associated with any particular genotype of HCV, the serum level of HCV RNA or the degree of fibrosis or inflammation on liver biopsy.

Treatment of Chronic HCV in Patients With PNAT

A large randomized, prospective controlled trial has evaluated the impact of treating patients with chronic HCV and PNAT with peginterferon alfa-2b and ribavirin.[5] In this study, patients were randomized to receive either 24 or 48 weeks of treatment or they were assigned to an observational arm and received no treatment. All treated patients received 800 mg of ribavirin (Figure 2-2). Overall, 52% of those patients treated for 48 weeks achieved a sustained virologic response (SVR). In patients with HCV genotype 1 who received 48 weeks of treatment the SVR was 40%. This declined to only 13% when the treatment duration was reduced to 24 weeks. Patients with HCV genotypes 2 and 3 had an SVR of 72% to 78% regardless of whether they were treated for 24 or 48 weeks. These rates for SVR were nearly identical to those observed for patients with elevated serum AT in

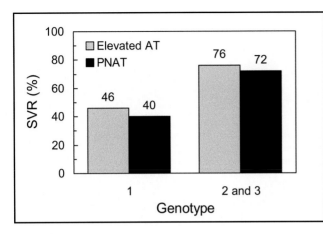

Figure 2-2. Comparison of SVR in patients with elevated serum AT and PNAT. Patients with genotype 1 were treated for 48 weeks. Patients with HCV genotypes 2 and 3 were treated for 24 weeks (Adapted from Fried M, et al. New Eng J Med 2002; 347:975-982 and Zeuzem S, Diago M, Gane E, et al. Peginterferon alfa-2a (40 kilodaltons) and ribavirin in patients with chronic hepatitis C and normal aminotransferase levels. *Gastroenterology.* 2004;127:1724-1732).

previous phase 3 clinical trials. It is therefore apparent that the HCV treatment paradigm, 48 weeks for patients with genotype 1 and 24 weeks for patients with genotypes 2 and 3, is also applicable for those patients with PNAT.

When patients with PNAT respond to peginterferon and ribavirin treatment, the serum AT declines. The mean value for serum AT for the patients enrolled in this study was 22 IU/L, and this declined to about 10 IU/L to 12 IU/L in those patients who became HCV RNA undectable during treatment. In patients who achieved an SVR, the serum AT remained at this low value. In contrast, patients who relapsed after peginterferon and ribavirin was stopped had a rise in serum AT back to the pretreatment baseline. This observation supports the claim that the "true" upper normal limit for AT is somewhere between 10 IU/L and 20 IU/L.

The frequency of AT flares during treatment with peginterferon alfa-2a in this study was nearly identical to that observed in the control group that was simply followed and did not receive peginterferon treatment. The level of increase in the AT during the flare was also similar. It is therefore apparent that peginterferon does not induce flares in patients with PNAT. Peginterferon treatment should therefore not be withheld from patients with a normal AT for fear that this might exacerbate HCV.

Many patients with chronic HCV report that they have a reduced quality of life. This is also true of patients with chronic HCV and PNAT.[6] Such patients report an increased frequency of fatigue and a decline in other health-related quality-of-life tasks on standard surveys compared to healthy individuals without HCV. Health-related quality of life improves in those patients with PNAT who achieve an SVR after being treated with peginterferon and ribavirin.

Summary

In summary, the majority of patients with chronic HCV and a PNAT have evidence of liver injury on liver biopsy and report a decline in their quality of life. Over time, at least 25% of these patients will develop an elevation in serum AT. Patents with PNAT respond to treatment with the same rates of SVR as other patients with chronic HCV. It was for these reasons that the second NIH Consensus Conference on HCV in 2002 recommended that patients with chronic HCV and PNAT should be evaluated in the same manner as all other patients with chronic HCV and be offered treatment if found to be an appropriate candidate.

References

1. Prati D, Shiffman ML, Diago M, et al. Viral and metabolic factors influencing alanine aminotransferase activity in patients with chronic hepatitis C. *J Hepatol.* 2006;44:679-685.
2. Shiffman ML, Stewart C, Hofmann CM, et al. Chronic infection with hepatitis C virus in patients with elevated or persistently normal serum alanine aminotransferase levels: comparison of hepatic histology and response to interferon therapy. *J Infect Dis.* 2000;182:1595-1601.
3. Hui CK, Belaye T, Montegrande K, Wright TL. A comparison in the progression of liver fibrosis in chronic hepatitis C between persistently normal and elevated transaminase. *J Hepatol.* 2003;38:511-517.
4. Puoti C, Castellacci R, Montagnese F, et al. Histological and virological features and follow-up of hepatitis C virus carriers with normal aminotransferase levels: the Italian prospective study of the asymptomatic C carriers (ISACC). *J Hepatol.* 2002;37:117-123.
5. Zeuzem S, Diago M, Gane E, et al. Peginterferon alfa-2a (40 kilodaltons) and ribavirin in patients with chronic hepatitis C and normal aminotransferase levels. *Gastroenterology.* 2004;127:1724-1732.
6. Arora S, O'Brien C, Zeuzem S, et al. Treatment of chronic hepatitis C patients with persistently normal alanine aminotransferase levels with the combination of peginterferon alpha-2a (40 kDa) plus ribavirin: impact on health-related quality of life. *J Gastroenterol Hepatol.* 2006;21:406-412.

DO ALL PATIENTS WITH CHRONIC HEPATITIS C VIRUS REQUIRE A LIVER BIOPSY?

Ramesh Ashwath, MD
Mitchell L. Shiffman, MD

Liver biopsy has long been utilized as a tool to both diagnose and or confirm the specific etiology of liver disease and to assess disease severity. The biopsy can be performed via percutaneous, transjugular, or laparoscopic techniques. The risk of complications associated with liver biopsy ranges from 0.5% to 2%. Bleeding complications occur most commonly in patients with thrombocytopenia or an elevation in INR and when a vascular mass is biopsied. In most large series, the risk of complications associated with diagnostic percutaneous liver biopsy in patients without laboratory evidence of cirrhosis was only 0.01% to 0.1%.[1] This is similar if not slightly lower than the risk of hemorrhage reported in patients who have a large poly removed during colonoscopy. It is therefore interesting that many gastroenterologists shy away from performing a liver biopsy, citing the high rate of complications, yet will gladly remove a large poly with the utmost of confidence.

Several systems have been developed to stage and grade the biopsy specimen. Most pathologists use the method they were taught during their training and are most comfortable with. Table 3-1 summarizes the most popular biopsy scoring systems. The precise numerical score is really not important. What is critical is that you understand how much inflammation (biopsy grade) and fibrosis (the stage) is present in the liver so that you can relate this to the patient in a manner he or she can understand. We tend not to fixate on the score but rather tell a patient he has either no, mild, moderate, or severe fibrosis (scarring) or cirrhosis. Patients tend to understand this much better.

The grade of the biopsy is important because it is the degree or intensity of inflammation that causes fibrosis progression. Thus, patients with no fibrosis and very mild inflammation have a very low rate of progression to cirrhosis. The majority of patients with mild inflammation and no fibrosis have persistently normal serum aminotrans-

Table 3-1

Summary of Liver Histology Scoring Systems

Description	Knodell Score	Metavir	Ishak	Scheuer
No fibrosis	0	0	0	0
Portal fibrosis	1	1	1 and 2	1
Portal fibrosis with septae extending outside of portal areas		2	2 and 3	2
Bridging fibrosis	3	3	3 and 4	3
Cirrhosis	4	4	5 and 6	4

ferases. Less than 20% of such patients develop any degree of fibrosis progression after 20 years. Patients in this category who do progress were probably understaged because of sampling error on the initial biopsy. In contrast, patients with significant degrees of inflammation will develop fibrosis progression. In general, there is a stepwise relationship between the severity of inflammation and the degree of fibrosis.

Are There Alternatives to Liver Biopsy?

The perceived risk and discomfort associated with liver biopsy have led to the development of several noninvasive methods to assess liver fibrosis. These include serum fibrosis markers, indexes that are calculated from standard blood tests and new imaging techniques. All of these noninvasive tests were developed in patients with chronic HCV and their utility in patients with other liver disorders, particularly cholestatic and noninflammatory liver disorders, remains unproven.

The AST/platelet ratio index (APRI) can be calculated from standard blood tests without additional cost.[2] AST is expressed as a function of the upper limit of normal (AST/upper normal value for AST × 100). As the degree of fibrosis increases, the AST increases with respect to the upper limit of normal and the platelet count declines. As patients develop advanced fibrosis and then cirrhosis, this ratio increases exponentially. Values greater than 1.5 are strongly indicative of advanced fibrosis or cirrhosis. In contrast, the test is unable to differentiate between patients with no or mild fibrosis. However, if the APRI index is increasing consistently over time, it is likely that fibrosis is progressing. The test was developed in patients with chronic HCV and it remains unclear whether this ratio correlates with fibrosis in other forms of chronic liver disease.

The Fibrotest was developed retrospectively by correlating the liver fibrosis score in patients with chronic HCV to a vast array of serum biochemical and hematologic markers.[3] Five markers (alpha-2-macroglobulin, haptoglobin, gamma-glutamyl transpeptidase, total bilirubin, and apolipoprotein A1) were selected though multivariate analysis. It is interesting to note that all of these biochemical tests are affected by inflammation and that none are precursors of fibrosis. These markers correlate with fibrosis because inflammation increases with the severity of fibrosis in patients with chronic HCV. It is unclear how these markers would perform in cholestatic and noninflammatory liver disorders.

The FibroScan is a specialized ultrasound unit that utilizes transient elastography to assess liver fibrosis.[4] Sound waves are sent into the liver and the speed at which these waves return to the transducer is related to the degree of liver stiffness, which increases with increasing fibrosis. The FibroScan device is not yet FDA approved. The accuracy of FibroScan appears to decline with obesity, either because the distance between the probe and the liver is increased by adipose tissue and this affects the elasticity measurements or because of the presence of coexistent NAFLD.

Each of these noninvasive tests of liver fibrosis can accurately differentiate patients with significant fibrosis (more than portal fibrosis) from patients with lesser degrees of fibrosis. However, neither of these tests can accurately differentiate patients with advanced bridging fibrosis and cirrhosis or differentiate patients with no fibrosis from patients with mild fibrosis. The ability to accurately identify patients with chronic HCV and no fibrosis and mild inflammation is important because these patients may never develop fibrosis progression and therefore may not require treatment.

How Does the Assessment of Liver Histology Help in Selecting Patients Who Require Treatment for Chronic HCV?

Many patients who find out that they have chronic HCV have risk factors that date back 10 to 30 years and, therefore, they have likely had chronic HCV for this long. If such a patient is found to have no fibrosis on liver biopsy, then HCV has obviously not caused any fibrosis to develop in 25 years. Such a patient is likely to have an excellent prognosis and is very unlikely to develop any fibrosis in the future.[5] Treatment is not necessary in these patients and will not alter the long-term prognosis, which is already excellent without treatment. However, if a patient is found to have any degree of fibrosis, he or she is likely to develop more fibrosis in the future and be at risk to develop cirrhosis. Such patients should be treated before they develop more advanced fibrosis since this is one factor that reduces the effectiveness of peginterferon and ribavirin therapy in patients with chronic HCV.

Many patients with chronic HCV are overweight and have type 2 diabetes mellitus and/or other factors associated with the metabolic syndrome. Such patients may have coexistent nonalcoholic fatty liver disease (NAFLD) or steatohepatitis (NASH). Several studies have clearly demonstrated that patients with chronic HCV and NAFLD or NASH have more advanced fibrosis and have a reduced response to peginterferon and ribavirin compared to patients without coexistent NAFLD. This information cannot be obtained by noninvasive liver fibrosis tests.

Table 3-2

Use of Liver Biopsy and Noninvasive Tests in Patients With HCV

	Liver Biopsy	*Noninvasive Tests*
Patient wants therapy regardless of liver disease histology	Not necessary	Not necessary
HCV genotypes 2 and 3	Not necessary	Not necessary
Patient unsure about therapy, but would take treatment if fibrosis present	Perform as first test or if noninvasive test suggests mild disease	Will require liver biopsy if result suggests mild fibrosis
Patients who were treated without liver biopsy but failed to achieve SVR	Perform as first test or if noninvasive test suggests mild disease	Will require liver biopsy if result suggests mild fibrosis
Patients with hemophilia who would only take treatment if fibrosis present	Requires factor replacement prior to procedure	Acceptable alternative
Incarcerated persons	Difficult and costly to perform	Acceptable alternative

Which Patients Should Undergo Liver Biopsy Prior to Initiating Treatment for Chronic HCV?

The potential uses for liver biopsy and the noninvasive fibrosis tests are listed in Table 3-2. It is not necessary to assess liver histology in all patients prior to initiating peginterferon and ribavirin treatment. Rather, liver histology should only be assessed when this information would aid in the management of the patient's liver disease. For example, if a patient with chronic HCV wants to be treated and would accept the adverse events associated with peginterferon and ribavirin even if a liver biopsy demonstrated no fibrosis, there is obviously no reason to perform a liver biopsy. For that matter, there is also no reason to perform any test to assess liver histology in such a patient. Most patients with chronic HCV genotypes 2 and 3 fall into this category because the rate of sustained virologic response (SVR) is high and treatment is for a shorter duration in most of these patients. However, such patients should have an assessment of liver histology if they fail to achieve an SVR. This would be necessary to determine whether the patient requires retreatment or can be safely monitored until more effective therapy is available.

If a patient with chronic HCV is worried about the adverse events of peginterferon and ribavirin and unsure if he really wants to receive treatment, then performing a liver biopsy is essential. None of the noninvasive tests can substitute for liver biopsy at this time since these tests cannot conclusively differentiate patients with no fibrosis from those with mild fibrosis. This is important because patients with mild fibrosis develop fibrosis progression and patients with no fibrosis may not. However, if a noninvasive test suggests that significant fibrosis is present, this information may be sufficient and a liver biopsy may not be necessary to confirm the exact degree of fibrosis. This is especially true if the noninvasive test suggests advanced fibrosis or cirrhosis since all of the noninvasive tests have excellent accuracy in this group. In contrast, if the noninvasive test suggests that mild fibrosis is present, a liver biopsy should be performed to determine just how mild this is and if no fibrosis is present.

Noninvasive tests of liver fibrosis are probably best utilized in specific populations where either the risk or cost of performing a liver biopsy is prohibitive. The most obvious patient populations in this group include those with hemophilia and patients who are incarcerated. Another potential use for noninvasive markers is to monitor for evidence of fibrosis progression in a patient with mild disease who either deferred treatment or failed to achieve an SVR during a previous course of treatment. However, these tests must be utilized with caution for this indication since no prospective data are currently available to inform us just how much of a change in the value of a noninvasive marker is significant and how much of a change in the noninvasive test needs to occur before this would be seen on liver biopsy.

Summary

Although the information provided by liver biopsy is generally useful, it is not necessary to perform this test in every patient prior to initiating treatment with peginterferon and ribavirin. Noninvasive tests of liver fibrosis are currently available. These are very accurate in identifying patients with advanced fibrosis or cirrhosis but have poor accuracy in identifying patients with no fibrosis who could easily defer or avoid HCV treatment. Patients who want to be treated for HCV even if they have no fibrosis do not need a biopsy or, for that matter, any other test to assess liver fibrosis. Probably the best use of noninvasive fibrosis markers is in those patients where liver biopsy is associated with increased risk and cost—the patient with hemophilia and the patient who is incarcerated.

References

1. Janes CH, Lindor KD. Outcome of patients hospitalized for complications after outpatient liver biopsy. *Ann Intern Med.* 1993;118:96-98.
2. Wai CT, Greenson JK, Fontana RJ, et al. A simple noninvasive index can predict both significant fibrosis and cirrhosis in patients with chronic hepatitis C. *Hepatology.* 2003;38:518-526.
3. Poynard T, McHutchison J, Manns M, Myers RP, Albrecht J. Biochemical surrogate markers of liver fibrosis and activity in a randomized trial of peginterferon alfa-2b and ribavirin. *Hepatology.* 2003;38:481-492.
4. Castera L, Vergniol J, Foucher J, et al. Prospective comparison of transient elastography, Fibrotest, APRI, and liver biopsy for the assessment of fibrosis in chronic hepatitis C. *Gastroenterology.* 2005;128:343-350.
5. Ghany MG, Kleiner DE, Alter H, et al. Progression of fibrosis in chronic hepatitis C. *Gastroenterology.* 2003;124:97-104.

How Often Should I Measure Chronic Hepatitis C RNA While Treating a Patient With Peginterferon and Ribavirin?

Mitchell L. Shiffman, MD

Achieving a sustained virologic response (SVR) following treatment of chronic hepatitis C virus (HCV) is the result of two separate processes. The first step is that the patient must respond to treatment and become HCV RNA undetectable. Patients who do not achieve a virologic response cannot achieve an SVR. The second step is to prevent relapse. Recent studies have clearly demonstrated that relapse is highly dependent upon how quickly and how long the patient first became and remained HCV RNA undetectable during treatment with peginterferon and ribavirin.[1] Recognizing the various patterns of virologic response and nonresponse and defining when a patient first becomes HCV RNA undetectable during treatment is therefore critical to maximize SVR. The various HCV RNA patterns that can be observed during treatment are illustrated in Figure 4-1.

Early virologic response is defined by a 2 log reduction in HCV RNA from the pretreatment baseline and/or being HCV RNA undetectable by treatment week 12.[2] Previous studies have clearly demonstrated that only those patients with an early virologic response (EVR) can achieve an SVR. Thus, patients with null response, the failure to achieve EVR, cannot possibly achieve an SVR. Traditionally, null response has been defined at treatment week 12. However, it is now apparent that null response may be recognized sooner. Patients who have no significant decline in HCV RNA at treatment weeks 4 and 8 really do not need to continue therapy for another month for null response to be recognized. Thus, monitoring HCV RNA at monthly intervals will allow the majority of null responders to be recognized sooner, and such patients can discontinue peginterferon and ribavirin earlier, thereby limiting the adverse events of treatment and reducing cost. Null response occurs in approximately 20% of patients with genotype 1 but only in about 3% of patients with HCV genotypes 2 and 3.

Figure 4-1. Response patterns observed in patients with chronic HCV during treatment with peginterferon and ribavirin.

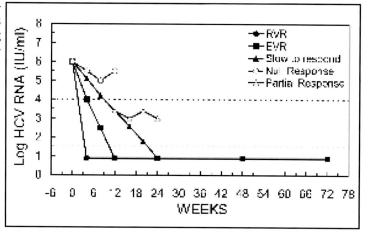

Another group of patients who fail to become HCV RNA undetectable are partial responders. Partial responders actually achieve an EVR. Unfortunately, the serum HCV RNA level that had initially declined by 2 logs from the pretreatment baseline within the first 12 weeks of treatment does not continue to decline. Rather, the serum HCV RNA level plateaus or stabilizes and remains positive at week 24. It is now well established that patients who remain HCV RNA positive at treatment week 24 will not become HCV RNA undetectable with further treatment and are therefore unable to achieve an SVR. Treatment should therefore be discontinued in partial responders at week 24. However, this cannot be done unless HCV RNA is assessed at this time point and these patients are recognized. Partial response occurs in approximately 15% of patients with genotype 1.

Overall, approximately 65% of patients with genotype 1 and 97% of patients with genotypes 2 or 3 become HCV RNA undetectable during treatment.[1,3] However, it has recently been recognized that the time at which these patients become HCV RNA undetectable is critical for achieving an SVR.

Patients who become HCV RNA undetectable within 4 weeks of initiating treatment are now referred to as having a rapid virologic response (RVR). These patients have a relapse rate of only 10%; their chance of achieving an SVR is 90% as long as they complete the proper duration of therapy—48 weeks for genotype 1 and 24 weeks for genotypes 2 and 3. Furthermore, the rate of SVR in patients with an RVR remains at 90% regardless of genotype, the serum level of HCV RNA prior to initiating treatment, liver histology, and the treatment received. Thus, patients with RVR who experience severe adverse events associated with treatment should reduce the doses of their medications, which will lessen these side effects and allow these patients to complete the proper duration of treatment. RVR occurs in approximately 15% of patients with genotype 1 and 66% of patients with genotypes 2 and 3. Recent studies have examined whether patients with RVR can reduce the duration of therapy to only 24 weeks or 16 weeks in patients with genotypes 1 and 2 or 3, respectively. Reducing the duration of therapy in such patients does yield high rates of SVR, around 80% to 85%. However, this is somewhat lower than what could be achieved with the standard duration of treatment. In our practice, we try to keep patients with an RVR on treatment for the proper duration whenever possible by reducing the dose of ribavirin and peginterferon if severe side effects occur.

Table 4-1

Rates of Relapse and Sustained Response in Patients With Chronic HCV During Treatment With Peginterferon and Ribavirin Based Upon Treatment Response Pattern

Week First Became HCV RNA Undetectable	Description	% of Patients	Relapse Rate, %	SVR Rate, %	Treatment Strategy
GENOTYPE 1					
4	Rapid response	15	10	90	Keep patients on treatment for 48 weeks even if have to reduce dose. If shorten therapy, SVR still very high
12	Early response	35	33	66	Complete 48 weeks of treatment
24	Slow to respond	15	55	45	Extend therapy to 72 weeks
Never	Null response	20	0	0	Stop treatment as soon as pattern recognized; 4 to 12 weeks
Never	Partial response	15	0	0	Stop treatment as soon as pattern recognized; 12 to 24 weeks
GENOTYPES 2 AND 3					
4	Rapid response	66	10	90	Keep patients on treatment for 24 weeks even if have to reduce dose. If shorten therapy, SVR still very high
After week 4	Early response	33	50	50	Consider extending therapy to 48 weeks
Never	Nonresponse	3	0	0	Stop treatment as soon as pattern recognized

Approximately 35% of patients with genotype 1 become HCV RNA undetectable between weeks 4 and 12.[1] These patients have a relapse rate of 33% or an SVR of 66% when treated for 48 weeks. However, the group that is very important to recognize are those with a "slow response." These patients do not become HCV RNA undetectable until treatment week 24 and this accounts for about 15% of genotype 1 patients. Patients who are "slow to respond" have a very high rate of relapse, 55% when treated for only 48 weeks, and an SVR of only 45%. However, recent studies have clearly demonstrated that if the duration of therapy is prolonged from 48 to 72 weeks, this high rate of relapse will be significantly reduced and this will lead to an increase in SVR.[4] At the present time it is unclear whether patients who become HCV RNA undetectable at treatment week 12 should also be treated longer than 48 weeks.[5] In our own practice, we only treat those patients who are slow to respond for 72 weeks.

Approximately 97% of patients with HCV genotypes 2 and 3 become HCV RNA undetectable with peginterferon and ribavirin. As noted above, approximately 66% of these patients achieve an RVR (HCV RNA undetectable at treatment week 4). The remaining 30% of patients with genotypes 2 and 3 have a high relapse rate, approximately 50%, and this reduces SVR in this group to only 50%.[3] Given the paradigms described above, such patients should be treated for longer than 24 weeks. However, no studies have yet demonstrated that this strategy, although logical, is effective in reducing relapse and improving SVR.

In summary, the sooner a patient becomes HCV RNA undetectable, the lower the relapse rate and the higher the SVR. The later a patient becomes HCV RNA undetectable, the higher the relapse rate and the lower the SVR. Patients with a null response can often be recognized prior to treatment week 12 and patients with partial response who remain HCV RNA positive at week 24 cannot achieve an SVR. Treatment should be discontinued in such patients as soon as these response patterns are characterized. Measuring HCV RNA at frequent intervals is therefore critical if we are to optimize the treatment of chronic HCV. This allows patients who are incapable of responding to treatment to be identified sooner so that treatment can be discontinued sooner. This also allows those patients who do respond to treatment to be better categorized so that the duration of treatment can be adjusted.

In our own practice, we measure HCV RNA at monthly intervals until the proper non-response pattern has been recognized and treatment is discontinued or until the patient becomes HCV RNA undetectable. If a patient with genotype 1 becomes HCV RNA undetectable after week 12, we prolong treatment to 72 weeks. If a patient with genotype 2 or 3 does not achieve an RVR, we prolong treatment to 48 weeks. We then measure HCV RNA at the end of therapy to document end-of-treatment response and 6 months off treatment to document relapse or SVR.

References

1. Ferenci P, Fried MW, Shiffman ML, et al. Predicting sustained virological responses in chronic hepatitis C patients treated with peginterferon alfa-2a (40 kD)/ribavirin. *J Hepatol.* 2005;43:425-433.
2. Sethi A, Shiffman ML. Approach to the management of patients with chronic hepatitis C who failed to achieve sustained virologic response. *Clin Liver Dis.* 2005;9:453-471.
3. Shiffman ML, Suter F, Bacon BR, et al. 16 vs. 24 weeks of peginterferon alfa-2a plus ribavirin for patients with HCV genotypes 2 or 3 infection. *N Eng J Med.* In press.
4. Sanchez-Tapias JM, Diago M, Escartin P, et al. Peginterferon-alfa2a plus ribavirin for 48 versus 72 weeks in patients with detectable hepatitis C virus RNA at week 4 of treatment. *Gastroenterology.* 2006;131:451-460.
5. Berg T, von Wagner M, Nasser S, et al. Extended treatment duration for hepatitis C virus type 1: comparing 48 versus 72 weeks of peginterferon-alfa-2a plus ribavirin. *Gastroenterology.* 2006;130:1086-1097.

WHEN A PATIENT RECEIVING PEGINTERFERON AND RIBAVIRIN THERAPY DEVELOPS ANEMIA SHOULD I PRESCRIBE EPOETIN ALFA OR REDUCE THE DOSE OF THE RIBAVIRIN?

Mitchell L. Shiffman, MD

Anemia is a common adverse event when patients with chronic hepatitis C virus (HCV) receive peginterferon and ribavirin. A decline in the serum hemoglobin by 2 g or more occurs in approximately 75% of these patients and up to 20% have a decline in hemoglobin of more than 4 g.[1] In large clinical trials the serum hemoglobin falls below 10 g/dL in approximately 20% of HCV patients during treatment; a decline in the hemoglobin to less than 8.5 g/dL occurs in about 5% of patients receiving peginterferon and ribavirin. Anemia significantly exacerbates the fatigue that many patients experience while receiving peginterferon and ribavirin, contributes to a significant reduction in quality of life, and is one of the most common reasons why patients discontinue HCV treatment.

Anemia in HCV patients receiving peginterferon and ribavirin results from a combination of ribavirin-induced hemolytic anemia and peginterferon-induced bone marrow suppression.[1] When patients are treated with either peginterferon or ribavirin alone, a 1-g decline in hemoglobin is typically observed. However, when these two agents are combined, the bone marrow suppression induced by peginterferon cannot accommodate for the ribavirin-induced hemolytic anemia, there is inappropriately low reticulocytosis, and the hemoglobin falls. Anemia is particularly severe in patients who have marginal iron stores. It is therefore essential that iron saturation and ferritin be assessed prior to initiating HCV treatment. If less than adequate iron stores are present, the initiation of treatment should be deferred until this is corrected with either oral or intravenous iron replacement.

The management of patients who develop anemia during treatment with peginterferon and ribavirin is an inexact science and remains controversial. This is because it has been very difficult to interpret the retrospective analyses performed on data obtained from large clinical trials and there have been no prospective studies evaluating different dose reduction strategies. In addition, the doses of peginterferon and ribavirin have been expressed as a percentage of the total cumulative dose that the patient should have received if no dose reduction had occurred. Thus, a patient may receive 80% of her medication through any number of dosing strategies (Table 5-1), and the impact of these on sustained virologic response (SVR) may be very different.

The first study to evaluate the impact of dose reduction demonstrated that SVR declined significantly when the cumulative doses of peginterferon and/or ribavirin declined below 80%.[2] However, the impact of dose reduction appeared to be confined to the first 12 weeks of treatment. No significant impact on SVR was observed in those patients who received less than 80% of their peginterferon and/or ribavirin when the dose modification occurred after week 12. In addition, reducing the doses of these medications appeared to have no significant effect on SVR in patients with HCV genotypes 2 and 3. Unfortunately, this study did not determine whether dose reduction alone, interrupting, or stopping these medications had a similar impact.

A more recent study evaluated the impact of deducing the ribavirin dose in patients with genotype 1 who remained on full-dose peginterferon throughout the entire 48 weeks of treatment.[3] This study also evaluated the impact of ribavirin dose in patients with different virologic response patterns (see Question 4). Ribavirin dose did not significantly affect virologic response, or the ability to become HCV RNA undetectable during treatment. In those patients with a rapid virologic response (HCV RNA undetectable by week 4 of treatment), the dose of ribavirin received had no impact on either relapse or SVR. In patients without rapid virologic response (RVR), SVR declined in only those patients who received less than 60% of their ribavirin doses.

The third study analyzed the impact of dose reduction in a genotype 1 nonresponder population undergoing retreatment with peginterferon and ribavirin.[4] This was also the only study to assess the impact of altering the peginterferon and ribavirin doses independently from each other and separate those patients who dose-reduced ribavirin from those who temporarily or prematurely stopped this medication. Lowering the dose of peginterferon below 80% led to a marked decline in both virologic response and SVR. In contrast, lowering the dose of ribavirin had no impact on either virologic response, relapse, or SVR as long as ribavirin dosing was not temporarily interrupted or prematurely discontinued. Permanently discontinuing ribavirin during the first 20 weeks of treatment led to a profound reduction in virologic response and SVR. Temporarily interrupting ribavirin dosing for greater than 7 consecutive days had a similar effect as permanent discontinuation.

In another study, patients with genotype 1 who became HCV RNA undetectable by week 24 were randomly assigned to discontinue ribavirin and remain on only peginterferon for the remaining 24 weeks of treatment or to stay on both medications for all 48 weeks of therapy.[5] Approximately 15% patients who stopped ribavirin developed breakthrough with reappearance of HCV RNA. These patients also had a significantly higher relapse rate. However, SVR was not affected by stopping ribavirin at week 24 in those patients who had an RVR and were already HCV RNA undetectable by week 4.

Table 5-1
Ways in Which a Patient Could Have Received 80% of His Medication

- 100% of dose for 24 weeks followed by 60% of dose for 24 weeks
- 100% of dose for 12 weeks followed by 73% of dose for 36 weeks
- 100% of dose for 1 week followed by 80% of dose for 39 weeks
- 100% of dose for 38 weeks followed by no medication for 10 weeks
- 100% of dose for 12 weeks followed by no medication for 3 weeks followed by 80% of medication for 33 weeks

---

A randomized placebo-controlled trial clearly demonstrated that the hemolytic anemia induced by peginterferon and ribavirin could be at least partially corrected by administering epoetin alfa.[6] The use of epoetin alfa in patients whose hemoglobin fell to below 12 mg/dL was associated with a marked improvement in quality of life and enabled 80% of patients to both remain on their starting ribavirin dose and to complete treatment. However, this study failed to assess the impact of epoetin alfa on either virologic response or SVR.

A randomized controlled trial has evaluated the ability of epoetin alfa, initiated at the onset of peginterferon and ribavirin treatment, to enhance SVR.[7] In this study, patients were randomly assigned to receive either peginterferon and ribavirin (P+R); peginterferon, ribavirin, and epoetin alfa (P+R+E); peginterferon; or a 200-mg higher dose of ribavirin and epoetin alfa. Although a significantly lower percentage of patients treated with P+R+E developed anemia and required ribavirin dose reduction, the SVR in this group was not significantly different than in the group treated with P+R. Patients treated with the higher dose of ribavirin (only 200 mg more per day) had a similar rate of virologic response as the groups treated with the standard dose of ribavirin. However, this group had a significant decline in the rate of relapse and therefore a significant increase in SVR compared to patients treated with the standard dose of ribavirin. This study strongly suggests that the routine use of eopetin alfa to treat anemia in patients with chronic HCV will not enhance SVR over that achieved by dose reduction. In addition, recent reports have clearly linked the use of epoetin alfa to an increased incidence of deep venous thrombosis and pulmonary embolus, placing these patients at risk without apparent benefit.

Several general observations should be taken from these studies that can provide insight into how symptomatic anemia could best be managed in HCV patients receiving peginterferon and ribavirin. These are summarized in Table 5-2. At our own center, we do not hesitate to lower the dose of ribavirin in response to a decline in hemoglobin but do so in 200-mg decrements, trying to keep the patient on as high a ribavirin dose as possible. Reducing the dose of ribavirin by only small amounts appears to have a minimal effect on SVR, especially in those patients who are already HCV RNA undetectable. In contrast, interrupting ribavirin dosing or prematurely discontinuing treatment even in patients who are HCV RNA undetectable leads to a significant reduction in SVR and

---

Table 5-2

Observations Regarding the Impact of Dose Reduction During HCV Treatment

- The primary role of peginterferon is to achieve a virologic response. Lowering the dose of peginterferon below 80% appears to reduce virologic response
- The primary role of ribavirin is to reduce relapse
- Reducing the dose of ribavirin has no impact on virologic response unless this medication is prematurely stopped
- The dose of ribavirin can be reduced without impacting SVR, especially in those patients with rapid virologic response (RVR) and in patients after they have become HCV RNA undetectable
- Interrupting or prematurely discontinuing ribavirin dosing leads to a significant decline in SVR. Every effort should be made not to miss ribavirin doses
- A higher initial starting dose of ribavirin appears to be associated with a lower relapse rate and higher SVR rate, even though patients who initiate treatment with higher doses of ribavirin require more frequent dose reduction
- Utilizing epoetin alfa to treat anemia in HCV patients receiving peginterferon and ribavirin has not been shown to enhance SVR
- Patients who develop profound anemia within the first 4 to 8 weeks after initiating HCV treatment with peginterferon and ribavirin cannot be successfully treated without epoetin alfa

---

should be avoided if at all possible. The only exception to this may be in persons with RVR.

Some HCV patients develop profound anemia with a decline in hemoglobin to under 8.5 g/dL within the first 4 to 8 weeks after initiating peginterferon and ribavirin. These patients cannot be managed by dose reduction alone and require epoetin alfa at the onset of therapy if they have any hope of responding to HCV treatment. In these patients the risk-benefit ratio of utilizing epoetin alfa may be justified. In all other HCV patients, reducing the dose of ribavirin and/or peginterferon appears to be a satisfactory way of handling anemia induced by these medications.

References

1. McHutchison JG, Manns MP, Brown RS Jr, Reddy KR, Shiffman ML, Wong JB. Strategies for managing anemia in hepatitis C patients undergoing antiviral therapy. *Am J Gastroenterol.* 2007;102:880-889.
2. McHutchison JG, Manns M, Patel K, et al. Adherence to combination therapy enhances sustained response in genotype-1–infected patients with chronic hepatitis C. *Gastroenterology.* 2002;123:1061-1069.
3. Reddy KR, Shiffman ML, Morgan TR, et al. Impact of ribavirin dose reductions in hepatitis C virus genotype 1 patients completing peginterferon alfa-2a/ribavirin treatment. *Clin Gastroenterol Hepatol.* 2007;5:124-129.
4. Shiffman ML, Ghany MG, Morgan TR, et al. Impact of reducing peginterferon alfa-2a and ribavirin dose during retreatment in patients with chronic hepatitis C. *Gastroenterology.* 2007;132:103-112.
5. Bronowicki JP, Ouzan D, Asselah T, et al. Effect of ribavirin in genotype 1 patients with hepatitis C responding to pegylated interferon alfa-2a plus ribavirin. *Gastroenterology.* 2006;131:1040-1048.
6. Afdhal NH, Dieterich DT, Pockros PJ, et al. Epoetin alfa maintains ribavirin dose in HCV-infected patients: a prospective, double-blind, randomized controlled study. *Gastroenterology.* 2004;126:1302-1311.

7. Shiffman ML, Salvatore J, Hubbard S, et al. Treatment of chronic hepatitis C virus genotype 1 with peginterferon and ribavirin and erythropoietin. *Hepatology.* 2007;46:371-379.

IS THERE ANYTHING I CAN DO TO IMPROVE THE CHANCE THAT AN AFRICAN AMERICAN WITH CHRONIC HEPATITIS C WILL RESPOND TO PEGINTERFERON AND RIBAVIRIN?

Mitchell L. Shiffman, MD

The spectrum of chronic hepatitis C virus (HCV) and its response to treatment appear to be somewhat different in African Americans compared to the general population of patients with this disease.[1] The prevalence of chronic HCV in the African American community is significantly greater than in Caucasians. Over 3% of all African Americans have chronic HCV, compared to only 2% of Hispanics and 1.5% of Caucasians. In addition, African Americans have a significantly higher percentage of HCV genotype 1 than is observed in other races; 97% of African Americans have HCV genotype 1 compared to 70% for all other persons in this country. Even the distribution of genotypes 2 and 3 appear to be altered in African Americans. In the general population, 30% of HCV patients have genotypes 2 and 3 and the distribution among these genotypes is roughly equal. In contrast, only 3% of African Americans with chronic HCV have genotypes 2 and 3 and nearly all African Americans with a non-1 genotype have HCV genotype 2. Genotype 3 accounts for only 0.5% of all HCV infections in African Americans.[2] The reason for the alteration in the distribution of genotypes in African Americans remains speculative. Clearly, African Americans are exposed to HCV through the same risk behaviors as persons of other races and must therefore be exposed to the same distribution of genotypes. It has therefore been hypothesized that the alteration in the distribution of HCV genotypes in African Americans is because persons in this racial group are able to spontaneously resolve nearly all acute exposures to genotype 3 and the majority of genotype 2 infections.

The natural history of chronic HCV also appears to be different in African Americans than in Caucasians. Although some studies have suggested that African Americans with chronic HCV have less severe inflammation and a lower prevalence of cirrhosis compared to the general US population with chronic HCV, this is not a universal finding. However, what is clear is that African Americans with chronic HCV and cirrhosis are at significantly increased risk for developing hepatocellular carcinoma (HCC). Large population-based studies have demonstrated that the risk of developing HCC is approximately 2-fold higher in African Americans compared with Caucasians for both men and women.[3] Furthermore, the survival of African Americans with HCC is significantly lower than in Caucasians. It is currently unclear whether this latter finding is secondary to delayed or lack of access to health care in the African American population or because African Americans have more aggressive and less curable HCC.

African Americans also respond far less well to interferon therapy than persons of other races. This observation was initially noted nearly a decade ago when standard interferon was administered 3 times weekly for treatment of chronic HCV. The SVR rate in African Americans with this treatment was only 2%, compared to 12% in Caucasians. The rate of SVR increased significantly when ribavirin was utilized along with standard interferon. However, this remained significantly lower in African Americans, only 11% when compared to Caucasians. Initially, this lower rate of SVR was attributed to the much higher percentage of genotype 1 in the African American population. However, 3 controlled clinical trials utilizing peginterferon and ribavirin have now documented that the SVR rates in African Americans with HCV genotype 1 are approximately 40% to 50% lower than observed in Caucasians of the same genotype.[4-6] The range in SVR observed for African Americans treated in these studies was 19% to 28% compared to 39% to 52% for Caucasians. In addition, a recent retrospective analysis has demonstrated that the SVRs in African Americans with genotypes 2 and 3 were only 52%, compared to 81% for Caucasian patients matched for genotype and various other parameters.[2]

The lower SVR observed in African Americans results from both an overall lower rate of virologic response and a higher rate of relapse. The patterns of virologic response were reviewed in Question 4. African Americans have a lower overall rate of early virologic response (EVR) and higher rate of null response. Within the category of EVR, the percentage of African Americans who do become HCV RNA undetectable at weeks 4, 12, and 24 is reduced compared to response rates observed in Caucasians (Figure 6-1). African Americans who do become HCV RNA undetectable tend to do so later during the course of treatment, and this slower rate of virologic response is associated with a higher relapse rate (see Question 4).

Several observations may help explain the slower and lower virologic response observed in African Americans. The ability of interferon to inhibit viral replication and increase HCV clearance is significantly reduced in African Americans. African Americans with chronic HCV have alterations in their cytokine profiles, less efficient T-cell responses to HCV antigens, and clear acute HCV infection less frequently than do Caucasians. Various aberrations in the immune response and differences in HLA alleles are also present in African Americans compared to Caucasians. Alternatively, recent data from several randomized controlled trials have demonstrated that the reduced SVR rate in African Americans is not secondary to differences in body weight, economic or envi-

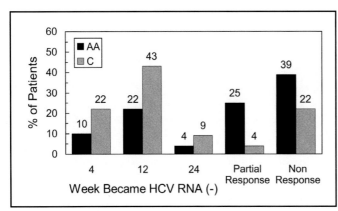

Figure 6-1. The percentage of African Americans and Caucasians who become HCV RNA undetectable at various time points during treatment, and those with partial and null response. (Adapted from Conjeevaram HS, Fried MW, Jeffers LJ, et al. Peginterferon and ribavirin treatment in African American and Caucasian American patients with hepatitis C genotype 1. *Gastroenterology.* 2006;131:470-477).

ronmental factors, or serum HCV RNA level. Interferon binds to its cell surface receptor equally well in African Americans as in Caucasians.

Based upon these data there are basically two strategies that can be utilized to enhance the effectiveness of interferon therapy in African Americans. One approach is to enhance the percentage of patients who respond to treatment and the second is to reduce the relapse rate. These strategies are summarized in Table 6-1.

Several studies have suggested that utilizing more interferon can enhance virologic response, but this benefit is likely confined to those patients with partial virologic response. Patients with partial response achieve a 2 log or greater decline in HCV RNA from pretreatment baseline but do not become HCV RNA undetectable. Partial responders as a group are somewhat responsive to interferon and may therefore become HCV RNA undetectable when higher doses of interferon are utilized. In contrast, it is unlikely that higher doses of interferon will affect virologic response in patients with null response. African Americans do have a higher percentage of null response. However, approximately 25% of African Americans exhibit a partial response and these patients may become HCV RNA undetectable when higher doses of interferon are utilized.

Another approach to enhancing SVR in African Americans is to reduce relapse. This can be accomplished in two ways: by utilizing more ribavirin and by treating patients for a longer duration. Two recent studies have demonstrated that utilizing a slightly higher dose of ribavirin, only 200 mg/day, can reduce relapse in both Caucasians and African Americans. Relapse is most common in those patients who become HCV RNA undetectable late during the course of treatment (see Question 4), and 2 studies have demonstrated that prolonging the duration of therapy from 48 to 72 weeks in these patients can reduce relapse. As a group, African Americans have a delayed response to treatment; therefore, continuing the duration of treatment from 48 to 72 weeks in those African Americans who become HCV RNA undetectable after week 4 would likely reduce relapse and enhance SVR.

At the present time none of these strategies has proven to be effective in enhancing SVR in African Americans with chronic HCV. However, based upon our current understanding of viral kinetics, response, and relapse, these strategies seem logical and worth implementing in motivated patients who have already demonstrated a virologic response to current treatment. In contrast, it is unlikely that African Americans with a null response would benefit from these strategies.

Table 6-1	
Strategies to Enhance SVR in African Americans	
Enhance response	Higher doses of peginterferon (ie, 360 mcg/week of peginterferon alfa-2a or 3.0 mcg/kg/week of peginterferon alfa-2b) or high-dose daily consensus interferon (9 to 15 mcg/d) in patients with partial virologic response If response occurs will need to extend treatment to prevent relapse (see prevent relapse)
Prevent relapse	Increase the dose of ribavirin by 200 mg/d or utilize weight-based ribavirin. This would have to be started at the onset of therapy or during retreatment. It is unlikely that increasing the dose of ribavirin in a patient already on treatment would provide the same effect Prolong the duration of therapy from 48 to 72 weeks in all African Americans except those with a rapid virologic response (HCV RNA undetectable at week 4)

References

1. Alter MJ, Kruszon-Moran D, Nainan OV, et al. The prevalence of hepatitis C virus infection in the United States, 1988 through 1994. *N Engl J Med.* 1999;341:556-562.
2. Shiffman ML, Mihas AA, Millwala F, et al. Treatment of chronic hepatitis C virus in African Americans with genotypes 2 and 3. *Am J Gastroenterol.* 2007;102:1-6.
3. Leykum LK, El-Serag HB, Cornell J, Papadopoulos KP. Screening for hepatocellular carcinoma among veterans with hepatitis C on disease stage, treatment received, and survival. *Clin Gastroenterol Hepatol.* 2007;5:508-512.
4. Muir AJ, Bornstein JD, Killenberg PG. Peginterferon alfa-2b and ribavirin for the treatment of chronic hepatitis C in blacks and non-Hispanic whites. *N Engl J Med.* 2004;350:2265-2271.
5. Jeffers LJ, Cassidy W, Howell CD, Hu S, Reddy KR. Peginterferon alfa-2a (40 kD) and ribavirin for black American patients with chronic HCV genotype 1. *Hepatology.* 2004;39:1702-1708.
6. Conjeevaram HS, Fried MW, Jeffers LJ, et al. Peginterferon and ribavirin treatment in African American and Caucasian American patients with hepatitis C genotype 1. *Gastroenterology.* 2006;131:470-477.

IS IT SAFE TO TREAT PATIENTS WITH CHRONIC HEPATITIS C AND CIRRHOSIS WITH PEGINTERFERON AND RIBAVIRIN?

Mitchell L. Shiffman, MD

Approximately 20% to 33% of persons with chronic hepatitis C virus (HCV) infection will develop cirrhosis. As discussed in Question 1, these patients are at risk to develop complications of chronic liver disease including hepatocellular carcinoma (HCC). As a result, the need for HCV patients with cirrhosis to be treated with peginterferon and ribavirin is far greater than for patients with mild chronic HCV. Furthermore, the overall cost benefit when a patient with cirrhosis achieves a sustained virologic response (SVR) is enormous, because this reduces future medical costs associated with complications of cirrhosis and liver transplantation.

Patients with cirrhosis have been included in nearly all of the large clinical trials designed to evaluate the efficacy of peginterferon with or without ribavirin. A specific study limited to patients with advanced fibrosis and cirrhosis was also conducted with peginterferon alfa-2a. All patients with cirrhosis included in these studies had normal liver function and no prior complications of cirrhosis and an imaging study of the liver demonstrating absence of any liver mass suspicious for HCC.

Patients with cirrhosis require periodic screening for evidence of HCC. Alfa-feto protein (AFP) is utilized by many gastroenterologists as one of the screening tests for this cancer. AFP is frequently elevated in patients with cirrhosis and this often raises concern for an underlying HCC.[1] All HCV patients with cirrhosis should be screened for HCC prior to initiating peginterferon and ribavirin. If an imaging study confirms that no suspicious lesions are present, then peginterferon and ribavirin can be initiated. A recent study has demonstrated that AFP declines when peginterferon and ribavirin are initiated, remains low while on treatment, and then elevates once this treatment is discontinued. In most cases the AFP returns to its pretreatment elevated level. However, in some patients the AFP will overshoot and rise above the previous baseline by a factor of 2-fold to 3-fold before gradually falling back to the pretreatment baseline. Such a dramatic rise in AFP after peginterferon and ribavirin are discontinued may raise concern that an HCC has developed and prompt the need for yet another liver imaging study. However, now that this phenomenon has been recognized it would not be unreasonable to monitor the AFP for several months after discontinuing peginterferon and ribavirin to see whether the AFP returns to its pretreatment baseline before requesting additional imaging studies.

Peginterferon suppresses bone marrow production of white blood cells and platelets, and the total white cell count, absolute polymorphonuclear count, and platelet counts all decline during treatment. In general, there is about a 20% decline in each of these cell lines. For this reason it was recommended that both the absolute polymorphonuclear and platelet counts be above certain minimum criteria to initiate peginterferon treatment. A polymophonuclear cell count of 1500/mm^3 has been utilized as a safe lower limit to initiate treatment. Although the package insert recommends that the dose of peginterferon be reduced if the neutrophil count falls below 750/mm^3, in our own practice we allow the absolute neutrophil count to fall to 500/mm^3 before reducing peginterferon. Studies have demonstrated that HCV patients with treatment-induced neutropenia are not at increased risk to develop significant bacterial infections and if patients do develop a bacterial infection while on peginterferon therapy they appear to mount an appropriate increase in the neutrophil count.[2]

According to the package insert, peginterferon alfa-2a can be safely initiated if the platelet count is above 70,000/mm^3 and above 90,000/mm^3 for peginterferon alfa-2b. However, these cut-off values for platelets are far above the safety level where the risk of bleeding increases due to thrombocytopenia, generally thought to be in the 20,000/mm^3 to 30,000/mm^3 range. In our own practice we feel comfortable initiating treatment with either peginterferon product as long as the platelet count is consistently above 50,000/mm^3 and will reduce the dose if the platelet count falls below 20 000/mm^3 to 25,000/mm^3.

HCV patients with cirrhosis have a lower SVR rate when treated with peginterferon and ribavirin than patients without cirrhosis. There are several reasons for this. Patients with cirrhosis respond to treatment at a slower rate than patients without cirrhosis. Most patients with cirrhosis who do respond to treatment become HCV RNA negative late during the course of treatment, between weeks 12 and 24, and therefore have a high relapse rate. As discussed in Question 4, continuing treatment for an additional 6 months, up to 72 weeks in patients with genotype 1 and up to 48 weeks for patients with genotypes 2 and 3, will reduce relapse and increase SVR. Patients with cirrhosis also have a higher incidence of adverse events, mostly related to cytopenias, and therefore need to discontinue treatment far more often than patients without cirrhosis. In addition, recent data from the NIH-sponsored HALT-C clinical trial has demonstrated that patients with cirrhosis have an innate lower rate of virologic response than patients without cirrhosis.[3] Despite these limitations, the benefits of treating patients with cirrhosis are potentially enormous. When a patient with cirrhosis does achieve an SVR, the risk of developing hepatic decompensation and the need for liver transplantation are significantly reduced; and if the patient does require transplantation at some point in the future, HCV will not recur.

One of the dangers in utilizing peginterferon to treat HCV patients with cirrhosis is hepatic decompensation. Patients with stable cirrhosis, normal liver function, and no prior episode of decompensation are at low risk to develop hepatic decompensation during treatment. However, patients with a previous episode of hepatic decompensation, variceal bleeding, ascites, or hepatic encephalopathy, or patients with Child-Pugh score greater than 6, are at increased risk to decompensate during treatment. Even if the prior complication had been treated and the patient is now clinically stable, the risk of hepatic decompensation during treatment with peginterferon still exists. As a result, we recommend that any patient with a prior episode of hepatic decompensation be first evaluated at a liver transplant center and considered a candidate for liver transplantation prior to initiating peginterferon treatment for chronic HCV. If such a patient is not a candidate for liver transplantation we do not consider he or she a candidate for treatment with peginterferon.

Treating HCV patients with cirrhosis and prior hepatic decompensation is a significant challenge. These patients are at significantly increased risk to develop severe neutropenia, thrombocytopenia, anemia, and typically experience significant systemic side effects and severe fatigue. As a result, an approach utilizing a low accelerating dose regimen (LADR) has been advocated.[4] According to this approach, patients are started on only 600 mg/d of ribavirin and either 90 mcg/wk or 0.5 mcg/kg/wk of peginterferon alfa-2a and alfa-2b, respectively. The doses of these medications are gradually increased over time. Both granulocyte colony stimulating factor (GCSF) and eopetin alfa (see Question 5) are also advocated to treat neutropenia and anemia, respectively. In the setting of cirrhosis, especially in patients with prior decompensation, nearly all patients will require growth factor support to be able to remain on treatment. Utilizing this strategy, approximately 25% of HCV patients with cirrhosis and a prior episode of hepatic decompensation can achieve an SVR.

Unfortunately, no good treatment for thrombocytopenia in HCV patients with cirrhosis receiving peginterferon currently exists. Interleukin-11 does stimulate platelet production and has been successfully utilized to treat chemotherapy induced thrombocytopenia. However, this agent causes significant fluid retention and patients with cirrhosis develop both edema and ascites from this agent. Interleukin-11 is therefore not recommended for use in these patients. Eltrombopag is an experimental agent that enhances platelet production and maturation and has been utilized in clinical trials to treat immune thrombocytopenia and thrombocytopenia secondary to cirrhosis and/or peginterferon. This oral agent appears to be highly effective, is currently entering phase 3 clinical trials, and should be available for general use within another 1 to 2 years. In the meantime, HCV patients with cirrhosis can be considered candidates for peginterferon therapy as long as the platelet count remains above 50,000/mm^3.

Table 7-1 summarizes recommendations regarding HCV treatment in patients with cirrhosis. HCV patients with stable cirrhosis and normal liver function should be considered candidates for treatment with peginterferon and ribavirin at the same doses as utilized for all other patients. Patients with a prior episode of hepatic decompensation can also be treated with peginterferon and ribavirin. However, these patients are at increased risk to develop hepatic decompensation and should therefore be evaluated at a liver transplant center prior to initiating treatment. If treatment is initiated in these patients with more advanced cirrhosis, a LADR approach utilizing GCSF and eopetin alfa to prevent neutropenia and anemia is typically required.

Table 7-1

Treatment of HCV Patients With Cirrhosis

Stable cirrhosis:
- Bilirubin, albumin, and INR all normal
- No previous complications of cirrhosis

Initiate treatment with peginterferon and ribavirin and usual doses and with usual strategy.
Extend therapy for an additional 24 weeks in those genotype 1 patients who become HCV RNA detectable between weeks 12 and 24. Extend therapy to 48 weeks in those genotype 2 and 3 patients who do not achieve rapid virologic response.

Prior episode of hepatic decompensation:
- Bilirubin, albumin, and INR currently normal

Consider evaluation at a liver transplant center prior to initiating HCV treatment. Treat with LADR protocol and utilize GCSF and epoetin alfa to prevent neutropenia and anemia.

Decompensated cirrhosis:
- Child-Pugh-Turcotte score > 8 and presence of ascites

Do not treat.

References

1. Di Bisceglie AM, Sterling RK, Chung RT, et al. Serum alpha-fetoprotein levels in patients with advanced hepatitis C: results from the HALT-C trial. *J Hepatol.* 2005;43:434-441.
2. Longman RS, Talal AH, Jacobson IM, Rice CM, Albert ML. Normal functional capacity in circulating myeloid and plasmacytoid dendritic cells in patients with chronic hepatitis C. *J Infect Dis.* 2005;192:497-503.
3. Everson GT, Hoefs JC, Seeff LB, et al. Impact of disease severity on outcome of antiviral therapy for chronic hepatitis C: lessons from the HALT-C trial. *Hepatology.* 2006;44:1675-1684.
4. Everson GT, Trotter J, Forman L, et al. Treatment of advanced hepatitis C with a low accelerating dosage regimen of antiviral therapy. *Hepatology.* 2005;42:255-262.

HOW OFTEN SHOULD I FOLLOW A PATIENT WHO HAD CHRONIC HEPATITIS C AFTER HE ACHIEVED A SUSTAINED VIROLOGIC RESPONSE?

Mitchell L. Shiffman, MD

Traditionally, a sustained virologic response (SVR) is defined as being hepatitis C virus (HCV) RNA undetectable 6 months after peginterferon and ribavirin are discontinued.[1] In the past it was unclear how long these patients remained HCV RNA undetectable or whether SVR was maintained long term and these patients were truly "cured" of HCV. No formal recommendations existed as to how these patients should be monitored. As a result, our practice, along with many other gastroenterologists, was to have these patients return once yearly to measure HCV RNA and to ensure that they remained an SVR.

To investigate the true meaning of an SVR, patients who were HCV RNA undetectable 6 months after completing treatment with peginterferon (with or without ribavirin) were enrolled in a long-term study to monitor HCV RNA over 5 years.[2] Nearly 1000 patients were enrolled in this study, including nearly 100 patients who were coinfected with HCV and human immunodeficiency virus (HIV) prior to receiving peginterferon and ribavirin. All of these patients were tested for HCV RNA at yearly intervals for a mean of 4.1 years; some patients were followed for as long as 7 years. During this time, over 99% of these patients continued to remain HCV RNA undetectable. Thus, for the first time, we can now safely say with confidence that patients who have achieved an SVR are cured of chronic HCV. Furthermore, these patients remained HCV RNA undetectable throughout the follow-up period regardless of the type of interferon they were treated with, whether or not ribavirin was utilized, regardless of genotype, serum HCV RNA level, and the severity of fibrosis prior to the initiation of treatment. Even those patients with cirrhosis who achieved an SVR continued to remain HCV RNA undetectable throughout the 5 years of follow-up and were cured of HCV.

Only 8 of the nearly 1000 patients enrolled in this study developed recurrence of HCV during the 5-year follow-up, and in at least some cases it appears that these patients may have acquired a new HCV infection by participating in high-risk behaviors. As a result, when patients achieve an SVR it may no longer be necessary to monitor these patients once yearly. We have now modified our practice somewhat and have these patients return at 1 and 5 years and no longer follow patients who have been HCV RNA undetectable for more than 5 years. Alternatively, patients could also be tested by their primary care referring physician. However, if you choose to refer your patients back to their primary care providers for long-term follow-up, it is important to ensure that they test for HCV RNA, not anti-HCV. Patients with an SVR will continue to be anti-HCV-positive for years, possibly even decades. Indeed, we have had patients who had an SVR over a decade ago referred back to our practice by their primary care provider because of a positive anti-HCV test but HCV RNA was found to still be undetectable.

Several centers have reported that some patients with a long-term SVR have very low levels of detectable HCV RNA in serum when assayed by ultrasensitive PCR techniques (low-level viremia). The meaning of these controversial findings remains unclear. Some investigators believe that this represents fragments of noninfectious and nonpathogenic hepatitis C virus that have remained in the patient. Others believe that this represents very low levels of HCV RNA replication and that such patients are at risk for future relapse. Whether this can explain at least some of the 0.8% relapse observed in the above-noted long-term follow-up study remains speculative. However, this observation provides a rationale to assess patients at some point after they achieve an SVR.

During the initial phase 2 and 3 clinical trials of interferon and peginterferon, a repeat liver biopsy was routinely performed 6 months after treatment had been completed. These studies demonstrated that patients with an SVR had less fibrosis compared to their pretreatment liver biopsy.[3] Whether fibrosis continues to resolve with time or completely resolves and the liver eventually returns to "normal" has yet to be demonstrated. In contrast, it remains controversial whether patients without an SVR derive significant histologic benefit from a single course of peginterferon.

Patients with cirrhosis represent an important group of patients with chronic HCV. These patients are at much greater risk to develop complications of cirrhosis and hepatocellular carcinoma (HCC) than patients without cirrhosis (see Question 1). In addition, the likelihood that these patients will achieve an SVR following treatment is significantly less than in patients without cirrhosis (see Question 7). Furthermore, in those patients who do achieve an SVR, the risk of hepatic decompensation and developing HCC is significantly reduced, but it is not eliminated.[4] In our own practice we have now seen 2 patients with cirrhosis develop HCC more than 5 years after achieving an SVR. These observations clearly demonstrate that it is imperative to continue to monitor patients with cirrhosis long term even after they have achieved an SVR. In our own practice, we assess these patients and screen for HCC at 6-month to 12-month intervals.

In summary, patients with chronic HCV who achieve an SVR are cured of chronic HCV. No formal recommendations as to how to follow these patients, if at all, currently exist. A rational recommendation for these patients is provided in Table 8-1. It is not unreasonable to ensure that each of these patients does in fact remain cured of HCV by assessing HCV RNA 1 and 5 years after completing treatment. Patients with chronic HCV and cirrhosis who achieve an SVR are also cured of HCV. However, they are not cured

Table 8-1

Recommendations for Monitoring Patients With Sustained Virologic Response

No evidence for cirrhosis	Check HCV RNA 1 and 5 years after completing treatment. If patient remains HCV RNA undetectable, no further follow-up necessary.
Evidence of cirrhosis	Check HCV RNA yearly after completing treatment. Assess liver function tests yearly after completing treatment. Screen for HCC at 6 2-month intervals.

of cirrhosis and remain at risk for developing complications of cirrhosis and/or HCC. Patients with cirrhosis must therefore be followed and screened for evidence of hepatic decompensation and HCC long term at regular intervals.

References

1. Lindsay KL. Therapy of hepatitis C: overview. *Hepatology*. 1997;71S-77S.
2. Swain MG, Lai MY, Shiffman ML, et al. Sustained virologic response resulting from treatment with peginterferon alfa-2a alone or in combination with ribavirin is durable and constitutes a cure: An ongoing 5-year follow-up. *Gastroenterology*. 2007;132(suppl 2):A741.
3. Poynard T, McHutchison J, Manns M, et al. Impact of pegylated interferon alfa-2b and ribavirin on liver fibrosis in patients with chronic hepatitis C. *Gastroenterology*. 2002 May;122(5):1303-13.
4. Imai Y, Kawata S, Tamura S, et al. Relation of interferon therapy and hepatocellular carcinoma in patients with chronic hepatitis C. *Ann Intern Med*. 1998;129:94-99.

SECTION II

VIRAL HEPATITIS B

WHICH PATIENTS WITH CHRONIC HEPATITIS B REQUIRE A LIVER BIOPSY?

Wei Hou, MD
Mitchell L. Shiffman, MD

Hepatitis B virus (HBV) infection is a significant global health issue that affects over 2 billion persons worldwide. In the United States, approximately 1.25 million persons have chronic infection and approximately 150,000 new infections are recorded each year. Individuals infected with HBV go through a series of serologic steps, which either results in spontaneous resolution of this virus and the development of protective hepatitis B surface antibodies (anti-HBs) or chronic HBV infection where hepatitis B surface antigen (HBsAg) persists in serum. Almost immediately after becoming infected, antibodies to hepatitis B core (anti-HBc) appear in serum, followed soon thereafter by HBsAg and then E-antigen. The E-antigen of HBV has traditionally been thought of as a marker of active viral replication. Over several weeks or months, the host immune response inactivates HBV and E-antigen becomes undetectable and is replaced by antibody (anti-E). This is followed by loss of HBsAg and the development of anti-HBs (Figure 9-1). The likelihood of spontaneously resolving HBV is directly related to patient age and whether jaundice occurred at the time of the acute infection. Thus, infants exposed to HBV vertically at birth rarely become jaundiced, only about 10% resolve the acute infection, and nearly 90% develop chronic HBV. In contrast, most adults develop acute icteric HBV and over 95% resolve this infection spontaneously.

Individuals who resolve acute HBV spontaneously and develop anti-HBs are immune and protected against reinfection from HBV. Over many decades, the level of anti-HBs in serum may decline below the level of detection. However, such persons typically remain positive for anti-HBc and anti-E. Administering a single dose of HBV vaccine acts like a booster in such individuals and results in the production of high-titer anti-HBs in serum.

Patients who develop chronic infection do not mount an appropriate immune response against HBV and remain HBsAg, E-antigen, and anti-HBc antibody positive (Figure 9-2).

Figure 9-1. Pattern of serum aminotransferse activity (AT) and serologic testing in a patients with acute HBV who develops spontaneous resolution.

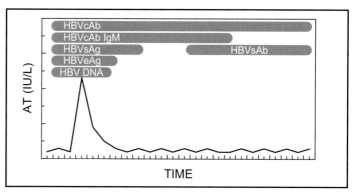

Such patients continue to have elevated serum liver aminotransaminases (AT), high levels of HBV DNA in serum, and active hepatitis on liver biopsy. After a variable period of time, many of these patients with chronic active HBV resolve E-antigen and produce anti-E, a step referred to as *seroconversion*. This process is typically preceded by an acute elevation in serum ALT and, in some cases, symptoms of acute hepatitis. Some patients may even become icteric. Patients who have had active HBV for many decades and developed cirrhosis prior to seroconversion are at risk of decompensation and liver failure when they serconvert. Following seroconversion, HBV becomes "inactive," replication of HBV DNA declines to very low levels, serum AT declines to the normal range, and liver inflammation resolves. Patients with inactive HBV may remain in this dormant state for decades. However, these patients remain at risk to "reactivate." This is why all patients with inactive HBV should be monitored at periodic intervals. Reactivation may occur spontaneously or in response to any process that suppresses the immune response, including chemotherapy, the use of immune suppressive agents, or coinfection with the human immune deficiency virus (see Question 16).

Viruses are prone to developing mutations and many variants of HBV are known to exist.[1] Mutations may alter specific proteins (antigens) produced by HBV in such a way that they are unrecognizable by current serologic tests. In some cases, antibodies produced by the host in response to mutant antigens may also not be recognized by current assays. A common mutant form of HBV is the "precore" mutant, where a single nucleotide substitution results in the formation of a stop codon along the open reading fame of the precore gene. This causes the E-protein to be shortened, no longer functional, and unrecognized by the E-antigen assay. However, patients with the precore mutant form of HBV have all other features of active HBV, including HBsAg, anti-HBc, elevated serum AT, high levels of HBV DNA in serum, and active hepatitis on liver biopsy. These patients should be referred to as having E-antigen–negative chronic active HBV. On average the level of HBV DNA in the serum of these patients is approximately 10-fold lower than observed in patients with E-antigen–positive chronic active HBV.

As outlined in Table 9-1, mutations may also occur in the surface and core genes of HBV. Although the hallmark of chronic infection with HBV is surface antigen, a mutation in this gene may yield a surface protein that cannot be recognized by the current assay. These patients are positive for anti-HBV core, have an elevation in serum AT, detectable HBV DNA in serum, and active hepatitis on liver biopsy but are HBsAg negative. Recognizing patients with active HBV and mutations in the surface gene may therefore

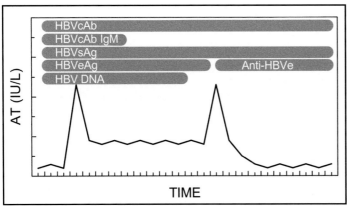

Figure 9-2. Pattern of serum aminotransferse activity (AT) and serologic tests in a patient with acute HBV who develops chronic active infection and then seroconverts to a chronic inactive.

Table 9-1

Mutations of HBV

	HBsAg	Anti-HBcore	E-antigen	HBV DNA
Wild-type virus	(+)	(+)	(+)	(+)
Precore mutant	(+)	(+)	(−)	(+)
Surface mutant	(−)	(+)	(+) or (−)	(+)
Core mutant	(+)	(−)	(+) or (−)	(+) or (−)

be a formidable challenge. In some cases, these patients may have anti-s, produced in response to a previous "wild-type" HBV infection. Mutations of the HBV core gene have also been reported. Such patients produce an abnormal core protein. In turn, the host either fails to produce an antibody against this protein or produces an antibody against HBcore that is not recognized by the current anti-HBcore assay. Such patients are recognized because they are positive for HBsAg and may have either active or inactive HBV.

As noted in Question 3, when the role of liver biopsy was discussed, in patients with chronic hepatitis C virus (HCV), a liver biopsy is also only necessary in patients with chronic HBV if the information gained by this procedure will affect disease management and, in particular, the need for treatment. In the case of chronic HBV, it is therefore best to assess the need for liver biopsy in relation to the serologic and biochemical status of the HBV infection.

Chronic HBV infection can be divided into 2 states as summarized in Table 9-2: active and inactive disease.[2] Patients with active HBV generally have an elevation in serum AT activity and serum levels of HBV DNA greater than 100 000 (1 × 10^5) IU/mL. On liver biopsy nearly all of these patients have active hepatitis with variable degrees of fibrosis. These patients may be either E-antigen positive or negative depending upon whether they

Table 9-2

Serology of Patients With Chronic HBV Infection

	Active HBV	*Gray Zone*		*Inactive HBV*
HBsAg	(+)	(+)	(+)	(+)
Serum ALT (IU/L)	Elevated	Elevated	Normal	Normal
E-antigen	(+) or (−)	(+) or (−)	(+) or (−)	(−)
Anti-E	(+) or (−)	(+) or (−)	(+) or (−)	(+)
HBV DNA (IU/mL)	>10^5	<10^5	>10^5	<10^5
Histology				
Inflammation	Active	Variable	Variable	None
Fibrosis	Variable	Variable	Variable	Variable

are infected with wild-type HBV or the precore mutant form of this virus. Almost all experts would agree that these patients should be considered candidates for treatment. At the other end of the spectrum are patients with inactive HBV. These patients tend to have normal serum AT and undetectable or low levels (<10^5 IU/mL) of HBV DNA. They are almost always E-antigen negative, anti-E positive and on liver biopsy they have no evidence of inflammation and in most cases no fibrosis. As a result, there is no reason why these patients require treatment for HBV.

Between these two extremes lies a grey zone of patients who do not fit into either of these two categories with discordant levels for serum AT and HBV DNA. One form of discordance is referred to as *immune tolerant* because the immune system does not appear to be mounting an effective immune response against HBV. On liver biopsy no inflammatory response against HBV-infected hepatocytes is apparent and as a result the serum AT is normal and serum HBV DNA is very high. It is unclear why the immune system appears to "tolerate" HBV in some patients. This phase of HBV may last for several months or decades. Treatment has not been advocated for patients with immune tolerance to HBV for several reasons. Without inflammation, fibrosis progression does not occur and as a result treatment yields no histologic benefit. However, a more important reason for not treating a patient in the immune-tolerant phase is that treatment is likely to be ineffective. It is currently believed that a viable immune response against HBV is required for treatment to be effective, and this appears to be true for both peginterferon and oral antiviral agents. Peginterferon works primarily by enhancing the immune response against HBV and if no immune response is present, peginterferon will be ineffective (see Question 10). Even very potent antiviral agents are unlikely to suppress HBV DNA to undetectable levels in patients without an immune response to HBV. As a result, the use of an oral antiviral agent in this setting is likely to promote resistance to the antiviral agent. For these reasons, all previous clinical trials evaluating either peginterferon or antiviral agents have excluded immune-tolerant patients. Performing a liver biopsy in these patients is often helpful to ensure that no ongoing inflammation is present and to confirm that the patient is indeed in an immune-tolerant state.

The other type of discordance is the patient with an elevated serum AT but low or undetectable HBV DNA. This pattern may be seen in patients with HCV or hepatitis D virus (HDV) coinfection because the coinfecting virus inhibits HBV replication (see Question 13). Alternatively, another cause for the elevation in serum AT, other than HBV, may be present histologically. Thus, liver biopsy is often essential in the patient with an elevated serum AT but low levels of HBV DNA.

Liver biopsy may also be helpful in many patients with mutations in the HBV genome. As noted above, the most common variant of HBV is the precore mutation. These patients cannot seroconvert to an inactive state either spontaneously or in response to treatment. The goal of HBV therapy in these patients is to suppress HBV DNA and this is typically a lifelong process (see Question 10). As a result, before committing a patient to lifelong treatment it is often important to document that treatment needs to be initiated at this time and should not be deferred. This is particularly true in young persons, where the lifelong risk of resistance needs to be balanced against the need to treat HBV. As a result, a liver biopsy may be useful in some patients with E-antigen–negative HBV. Performing a liver biopsy and confirming active HBV infection through immunohistochemical staining of liver tissue is also helpful in patients with atypical serologic HBV testing. This is most commonly observed in patients with mutations in the surface or core genes or in patients who are also infected with HCV, HDV, or human immunodeficiency virus (HIV).

In summary, a liver biopsy is not necessary in patients with classic E-antigen–positive or E-antigen–negative HBV as long as no absolute or relative contraindications to treatment exist. Similarly, a liver biopsy is not indicated for patients with inactive HBV since such patients do not require therapy. However, we find that a liver biopsy is extremely useful in those patients who fall outside these classic criteria and in patients with unusual mutations of the HBV genome. A liver biopsy is also useful in young patients with E-negative chronic active HBV since this carries with it a lifelong risk of resistance. These issues will be discussed in more detail in Questions 10 through 12.

References

1. Baumert TF, Barth H, Blum HE. Genetic variants of hepatitis B virus and their clinical relevance. *Minerva Gastroenterol Dietol.* 2005;51:95-108.
2. Keeffe EB, Dieterich DT, Han SH, et al. A treatment algorithm for the management of chronic hepatitis B virus infection in the United States: an update. *Clin Gastroenterol Hepatol.* 2006;4:936-962.

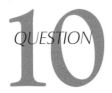
HOW DO I DECIDE WHICH MEDICATION TO UTILIZE IN A PATIENT WITH HEPATITIS B VIRUS?

Mitchell L. Shiffman, MD

Several medications are currently available for the treatment of chronic hepatitis B virus (HBV) infection (Table 10-1). These can be divided into 2 basic categories; interferons and oral antiviral agents. Both standard interferon alfa-2b and peginterferon alfa-2a have been shown to be effective and are approved by the Food and Drug Administration (FDA).[1,2] Four oral antiviral agents have also been FDA approved;[3-8] tonofovir is also known to be effective against HBV and will likely be approved within the near future. When considering which of these agents to utilize in a patient with chronic HBV it is first necessary to consider the primary and secondary goals of therapy. These goals are different depending upon the serologic status and genotype of HBV, the race, nationality, and age of the patient, and the degree of liver fibrosis present on liver biopsy. As opposed to patients with chronic hepatitis C virus (HCV), chronic HBV exists in two basic forms: active disease and inactive disease. Patients with inactive disease do not require treatment. Patients with acute icteric HBV also do not require treatment since over 90% of these patients will resolve this infection spontaneously and develop protective anti-HBsurface. The various serologic patterns of chronic HBV, how to utilize these serologic markers to differentiate active from inactive HBV, and which patients may require liver biopsy to aid in this decision were discussed in Question 9.

Approximately half of the estimated 1.25 million persons with chronic HBV in the United States have either immigrated to this country from Southeast Asia or Indochina where HBV is endemic and acquired vertically or are first-generation Americans with mothers who immigrated from this area of the world. The remaining patients with chronic HBV are immigrants from eastern Europe or Africa who may have also acquired HBV either vertically or shortly after birth or are persons who acquired HBV through percutaneous or sexual exposures as young adults.

Table 10-1

Agents Utilized for the Treatment of E-Antigen Positive Chronic HBV

	Duration of Treatment, Weeks	Normal ALT, %	HBV DNA Undetectable, %	Sero Conversion, %
Standard interferon	16	25	25	25
Peginterferon	48	41	14	32
Lamivudine	48	60	36	18
Adefovir	48	48	21	12
Entecovir	48	68	67	21
Telbivudine	48	77	60	22

Data obtained from Lau et al,[1] Marcellin et al,[2,3] Hadziyannis et al,[4,5] Chang et al,[6] Lai et al,[7] and Hoofnagle et al.[8]

Several genotypes of HBV, A through E, exist. Genotype is one of the most important factors associated with seroconversion during treatment. Slightly more than 50% of patients with E-antigen–positive HBV and genotype A will seroconvert when treated with peginterferon. Patients with genotype A are almost always non-Asian. In contrast, nearly all Asians with chronic HBV are genotypes C or D. The rate of seroconversion in patients with non-A genotypes is only about 30%.

The E-Antigen–Positive Patient

The primary goal of treatment in a patient with E-antigen–positive chronic active HBV is E-antigen seroconversion. This is associated with both the loss of E-antigen and the appearance of anti-E. If this occurs, several secondary goals are also realized. These include a decline in serum HBV DNA to either very low or undetectable levels, normalization in serum alanine aminotransferase (ALT), improvement in liver histology, and a reduced risk of hepatocellular carcinoma (HCC).

Either interferon, peginterferon, or an oral antiviral agent can be utilized to treat E-antigen–positive chronic HBV. The benefits of interferon are that the treatment is finite and the response is absolute. Peginterferon is administered at a dose of 180 mcg/wk for 48 weeks and seroconversion occurs either during or within 6 months of discontinuing this treatment or it does not occur. There is no apparent benefit to continuing treatment longer. Indeed, a similar seroconversion rate was observed with 5 million units of standard interferon administered every day for 16 weeks. As a result, a shorter duration and lower

Table 10-2

Agents Utilized for the Treatment of E-antigen–Negative Chronic HBV*

	Normal ALT, %	HBV DNA Undetectable, %	Resistance at 2 Years*, %
Peginterferon	59	19	N/A
Lamivudine	71	72	42
Adefovir	72	51	3
Entecovir	78	90	0 or 9[†]
Telbivudine	74	88	22

*Data obtained from Lau et al,[1] Marcellin et al,[2,3] Hadziyannis et al,[4,5] Chang et al,[6] Lai et al,[7] and Hoofnagle et al.[8]
[†]Resistance data are for both E-Ag–positive or E-Ag–negative patients. Data for entecovir are 0% in treatment of naive patients and 9% in patients with prior lamivudine resistance.

dose of peginterferon are currently being evaluated. In patients with seroconversion this response is long lasting. The downside of peginterferon is that it is administered by sub-cutaneous injection and is associated with flu-like side effects. However, compared to patients with chronic HCV who also take ribavirin with peginterferon, the adverse events reported by patients with chronic HBV appear to be significantly less severe. As noted above, the highest rates of E-antigen seroconversion, slightly more than 50%, occurs in patients with HBV genotype A. In patients with all other genotypes, the seroconversion rate is only about 30%. If seroconversion does not occur, serum HBV DNA and ALT either remain or return to their pretreatment baseline.

Patients with cirrhosis are not good candidates for peginterferon therapy. One of the dangers of peginterferon treatment is that patients may flare and develop marked eleva-tions in serum ALT at the time of seroconversion. Although this has minimal risk in a patient without cirrhosis, patients with cirrhosis and marginal hepatic reserve are at increased risk to decompensate and develop liver failure during a flare.

The primary goal of therapy when utilizing an oral antiviral agent to treat E-anti-gen–positive chronic HBV is also seroconversion. However, each of the antiviral agents is less effective at achieving this goal within the first year compared to peginterferon. In contrast, all of the oral antiviral agents are more effective at suppressing HBV DNA and achieving the secondary goals of treatment than is peginterferon. Each of the oral antiviral agents differ somewhat in overall potency. This affects the speed at which HBV DNA declines during treatment and ultimately the percentage of patients who become HBV DNA undetectable (Table 10-2). Of the currently available oral antiviral agents, ente-covir is the most potent. Approximately 66% of patients with E-antigen–positive chronic HBV become HBV DNA undetectable during the first year of treatment with entecovir.

Unfortunately, this does not translate into a higher rate of seroconversion, which occurs in only 12% to 20% with the various oral antiviral agents. Adefovir does lower HBV DNA at a slower rate than entecovir. However, this decline is steady, consistent, and continues over several years. Thus, the percentage of patients who become HBV DNA undetectable with adefovir increases each year, as does the rate of E-antigen seroconversion. After 3 years of treatment with adefovir, 44% of patients have achieved seroconversion, a value similar to that observed after 1 year of peginterferon. Antiviral agents are extremely popular with patients because they are taken orally and have virtually no side effects. Their main limitation is the development of resistant mutations and this could affect the patient's ability to respond to other medications (see Question 12).

In our own practice we recommend that all non-Asians with E-antigen–positive chronic HBV be tested for genotype. We do not test for genotype in Asians since it is extremely unlikely that the A genotype would be found. Unless a patient has evidence of cirrhosis, patients with genotype A are encouraged to be treated with peginterferon because they have such a high rate of serconversion with just 24 to 48 weeks of treatment. We also encourage young patients regardless of genotype, race, or nationality, and especially those with mild disease on liver biopsy, to be treated with peginterferon. If these patients fail to seroconvert with peginterferon, we then reassess their need for treatment, especially if they are young. This limits the exposure of these patients to oral antiviral agents and reduces their lifetime risk of developing resistant mutations to these medications. Those patients who have significant liver injury and either failed to seroconvert or deferred treatment with peginterferon are started on either adefovir of entecovir and their virologic response is monitored at 3-month intervals. We favor these agents because of their low rate of resistance. Treatment is continued indefinitely or until after seroconversion has occurred (see Question 11).

The E-antigen–Negative Patient

Patients with E-antigen–negative active HBV cannot seroconvert. As a result, the primary goal of treatment in these patients is viral suppression. All of the oral antiviral agents are effective in suppressing HBV DNA and several studies have demonstrated that this is associated with secondary gains, which include normalization in serum ALT, improvement in liver histology, and a reduced risk of HCC. Discontinuing antiviral therapy is associated with recurrent viremia and the development of resistant mutations. Reinstating treatment is possible but may be less effective if a resistance mutation has emerged. Thus, once treatment with an oral antiviral agent is initiated, it should be continued lifelong and not stopped even for brief periods of time (see Question 11). It is therefore imperative that the E-antigen status of the patient has been documented and the pros and cons of initiating oral antiviral therapy be carefully considered before treatment is initiated. In our own practice we would try to avoid initiating antiviral therapy in young persons with E-antigen–negative active HBV, especially in those patients with only modest elevations in serum HBV DNA and mild fibrosis on liver biopsy, because of the lifetime risk of noncompliance and the development of resistant mutations. However, if significant liver injury were present, we would not hesitate to start the patient on either adefovir or entecovir and monitor HBV DNA at 3-month intervals. We favor these agents because they have the lowest rate of resistance. Once the patient becomes HBV DNA undetectable, the frequency of monitoring can be reduced to once every 6 months.

Peginterferon has also been utilized in patients with E-antigen–negative active HBV. Initially, this was not thought to be a very attractive treatment for this form of HBV because seroconversion cannot occur and the majority of patients simply develop recurrence of HBV after treatment is discontinued. However, it has recently been demonstrated that about 30% of patients will respond to 48 weeks of peginterferon treatment, become HCV RNA undetectable, and remain in an "inactive" state for several years after treatment has been discontinued.

References

1. Lau GK, Piratvisuth T, Luo KX, et al. Peginterferon Alfa-2a, lamivudine, and the combination for HBeAg-positive chronic hepatitis B. *N Engl J Med*. 2005;352:2682-2695.
2. Marcellin P, Lau GK, Bonino F, et al. Peginterferon alfa-2a alone, lamivudine alone, and the two in combination in patients with HBeAg-negative chronic hepatitis B. *N Engl J Med*. 2004;351:1206-1217.
3. Marcellin P, Chang TT, Lim SG, et al. Adefovir dipivoxil for the treatment of hepatitis B e antigen-positive chronic hepatitis B. *N Engl J Med*. 2003;348:808-816.
4. Hadziyannis SJ, Tassopoulos NC, Heathcote EJ, et al. Adefovir dipivoxil for the treatment of hepatitis B e antigen-negative chronic hepatitis B. *N Engl J Med*. 2003;348:800-807.
5. Hadziyannis SJ, Tassopoulos NC, Heathcote EJ, et al. Long-term therapy with adefovir dipivoxil for HBeAg-negative chronic hepatitis B. *N Engl J Med*. 2005;352:2673-2681.
6. Chang TT, Gish RG, de Man R, et al. A comparison of entecavir and lamivudine for HBeAg-positive chronic hepatitis B. *N Engl J Med*. 2006;354:1001-1010.
7. Lai CL, Shouval D, Lok AS, et al. Entecavir versus lamivudine for patients with HBeAg-negative chronic hepatitis B. *N Engl J Med*. 2006;354:1011-1020.
8. Hoofnagle JH, Doo E, Liang TJ, Fleischer R, Lok AS. Management of hepatitis B: summary of a clinical research workshop. *Hepatology*. 2007;45:1056-1075.

CAN I EVER STOP TREATMENT IN A PATIENT WITH CHRONIC HEPATITIS B RECEIVING AN ORAL ANTIVIRAL AGENT?

Wei Hou, MD
Mitchell L. Shiffman, MD

Oral antiviral agents are very effective in the treatment of both E-antigen–positive and E-antigen–negative chronic active hepatitis B virus (HBV).[1-3] These agents act by suppressing HBV replication and lowering the serum level of HBV DNA. The ultimate goal is to render the patient HBV DNA undetectable by a sensitive polymerase chain reaction (PCR) assay. Whether this goal can be achieved and how long this will require after treatment is initiated is dependent upon the serum level of HBV DNA at the time treatment is initiated, the potency of the antiviral agent utilized, and the resistance rate associated with the particular antiviral agent. In general, the higher the level of HBV DNA, the longer it will take the patent to become HBV DNA undetectable regardless of the specific antiviral agent utilized. In addition, a very high level of HBV DNA at baseline (>100 million IU/mL) is associated with a lower likelihood that the patient will become HBV DNA undetectable and a higher likelihood that a resistant strain of HBV will emerge at some time during treatment. This is of greatest concern in E-antigen–positive patients where the level of HBV DNA is usually 10 to 100 times higher than in E-antigen–negative patients. The highest levels of HBV DNA are often seen in those E-antigen–positive patients with "immune tolerance" (see Questions 9 and 10). This is associated with normal serum aminotransferases (AT) and no significant inflammation on liver histology. Most experts would agree that these particular patients have a low likelihood of becoming HBV DNA undetectable are at high risk to develop resistance and should therefore be monitored but not be treated.

Four oral antiviral agents are currently approved by the Food and Drug Administration for the treatment of chronic HBV.[1,2] The effectiveness of these agents were summarized in Question 10 (see Tables 10-1 and 10-2). Of these agents, entecovir is the most potent, is associated with the most rapid decline in serum HBV DNA level, and has the highest percentage of patients becoming HBV DNA undetectable after 1 year of treatment. Lamivudine and telbivudine are also very effective in suppressing HBV DNA. However, both of these agents have a higher rate of selecting for resistant HBV mutations. Lamivudine was the first of the oral antiviral agents available for treatment of chronic HBV, has the longest track record, and its resistance profile is well characterized. Approximately 25% of patients treated with lamivudine develop resistance after just 1 year and this increases to 70% after 4 years of continuous treatment. Telbivudine is the most recent of the 4 oral anti-HBV drugs. After 1 year a resistance rate of approximately 22% has been observed to date. This is likely to increase with long-term use. Adefovir dipivoxil lowers HBV DNA at a somewhat slower rate than either of the other antiviral agents. Despite this, HBV DNA continues to decline with continued treatment in the great majority of patents and no resistance has been observed with this agent within the first year. After 4 years of continuous therapy with adefovir, resistant mutations emerged in only 8% of patients.

The indications to initiate therapy in patients with chronic HBV were discussed in Questions 9 and 10. The endpoints of treating chronic HBV are dependent upon the E-antigen status of the patient prior to initiating treatment. Since spontaneous conversion of E-antigen chronic active HBV can occur at any time it is imperative that the E-antigen status and the serum HBV DNA level of the patient be defined immediately before treatment is initiated, even in those patients where this was assessed several months previously.

The E-Antigen–Positive Patient

The ultimate goal of treatment in a patient with E-antigen–positive chronic active HBV is seroconversion. However, this cannot occur until a patient has first become HBV DNA undetectable. The response rate observed with oral antiviral therapy in patients with E-antigen–positive chronic HBV was summarized in Question 10. In general, 20% to 66% of patients will normalize serum AT activity and become HBV DNA undetectable during treatment. Despite this, oral antiviral agents are less effective in the short term at achieving seroconversion than peginterferon. However, in those patients who do become and remain HBV DNA undetectable the rate of seroconversion appears to increase stepwise over time. The only agent with long-term seroconversion data available to date is adefovir dipivoxil. In these studies, 13% of patients lost E-antigen after 1 year of treatment and this increased to 23% after 2 years and 44% after 3 years. Thus, the rate of seroconversion after 3 years of treatment with adefovir appeared to be similar to that achieved with a limited course of peginterferon.

Once E-antigen seroconversion has occurred in a patient being treated with an oral antiviral agent this treatment should be continued for an additional 6 months. Data to support this recommendation come from a single study where patients with E-antigen–positive HBV were treated with adefovir dipivoxil for 1 year. All patients who seroconverted during treatment were then monitored for a mean of 3 additional years for evidence of seroreversion and recurrence of HBV DNA. Forty-one of 45 patients in this study (91%) remained E-antigen negative, anti-E positive, and HBV DNA undetectable. The 4 patients who seroreverted and again became E-antigen and HBV DNA positive discontinued adefovir only 12 to 16 weeks after seroconversion.

Based upon these observations we have adopted the following algorithm for monitoring patients with E-antigen–positive chronic active HBV who are treated with an oral antiviral agent. At the time treatment is initiated we repeat testing for E-antigen and anti-E, HBV DNA, and AT activity. These patients are then monitored 1 and 3 months after treatment is initiated to assess for adverse events and then at 3-month intervals thereafter if treatment is well tolerated. At each visit serum AT activity and HBV DNA are assessed. Once patients become HBV DNA undetectable, E-antigen status is assessed at each visit. If E-antigen becomes undetectable, both E-antigen and anti-E are then assessed at subsequent visits. Six months after both E-antigen has resolved and anti-E has appeared, treatment can be safely discontinued. In most patients this will require several years of treatment.

Seroconversion is not a cure for HBV. Rather, the patient has converted from an active to an inactive state of the disease. Approximately 5% of these patients may lose HBsAg and develop anti-S. It remains unclear whether the percentage of patients who achieve S-antigen seroconversion following treatment with an oral antiviral agent increases over time as is observed following treatment with interferon. Since the majority of patients remain HBsAg positive, periodic monitoring and screening for hepatocellular carcinoma (HCC) is therefore necessary. During each of these visits we also assess for S-antigen and if this becomes undetectable we then also assess for anti-S at subsequent visits (Table 11-1).

The E-Antigen–Negative Patient

The goal of treating patients is to suppress HBV DNA to undetectable levels. In general, patients with E-antigen–negative chronic HBV have a serum HBV DNA level that is 10-fold to 100-fold lower than patients who are E-antigen positive. As a result, the likelihood of becoming HBV-DNA undetectable with oral antiviral therapy is higher in the E-antigen negative than for the E-antigen–positive patient. In general, 50% to 90% of E-antigen–negative patients with chronic active HBV will normalize serum AT activity and become HBV DNA undetectable during treatment with an oral antiviral agent (see Question 10). However, patients with E-antigen–negative chronic active HBV cannot seroconvert. As a result, once a decision is made to initiate treatment this should be continued lifelong. Discontinuing treatment is associated with a rise in HBV-DNA (Figure 11-1).

Patients who do not become HBV DNA undetectable with an oral antiviral agent are at risk to develop both disease progression and viral resistance. As a result, patients who remain HBV DNA positive without any further decline in HBV DNA 6 to 12 months after treatment was initiated should either be switched to an alternative oral agent or have a second agent added to the treatment regimen. When combing oral antiviral agents it is imperative that their site of action be different. Lamivudine, entecovir, and telbivudine all inhibit HBV replication at the same site of action. Thus, these agents should not be combined. Only adefovir acts at a different site to inhibit HBV replication and can be combined with any of the other three agents.

Patients With Cirrhosis

Patients with cirrhosis, regardless of E-antigen status, require a different approach than HBV patients without cirrhosis. Patients with chronic HBV and cirrhosis have an increased risk of developing HCC and therefore every effort should be made to keep HBV

Table 11-1

Biochemical, Virologic, and Serologic Testing During Treatment of E-antigen–Positive Chronic HBV

Time	AT*	HBV DNA	E-Ag	anti-E	sAg	anti-s
Baseline	x	x	x	x	1†	1†
Month 1	x	x				
Month 3	x	x				
Every 3 months	x	x				
If HBV DNA remains positive with no further decline after 6 to 12 months consider adding a second or switching to an alternate agent						
Continue monitoring every 3 months	x	x				
After HBV DNA becomes undetectable						
Every 3 months	x	2‡	x			
After E-antigen becomes undetectable						
Every 3 months	x	2‡	x	x		
After anti-E becomes detectable						
Every 3 months	x	2‡	x	x	x	
After anti-E has been undetectable for 6 months. Treatment can be discontinued except in patients with cirrhosis						
Every 6-12 months	x	2‡	3§	3§	x	
After s-antigen becomes unde-tectable						
Every 6-12 months	x	3§	3§	3§	x	x
After s-antigen becomes posi-tive	4‖	4‖	4‖	4‖	4‖	4‖

*AT indicates aminotransferases.
†sAg and anti-s need not be repeated if this is documented within the past 6 to 12 months.
‡HBV DNA should continue to be monitored to ensure that a resistant form does not emerge.
§It would be highly unusual for HBV DNA to recur, E-antigen to again become positive, or anti-E to become negative more than 6 months after seroconversion. These tests do not need to be repeated at every visit. However, it would not be unreasonable to perform these tests every 1 to 2 years, especially in patients with cirrhosis.
‖It remains unclear how patients with s-antigen seroconversion should be monitored. It would be reasonable to assess such patients every 1 to 2 years. Patients with cirrhosis should be monitored more frequently.

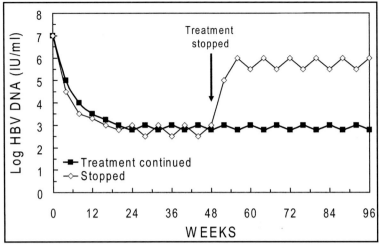

Figure 11-1. Effect of discontinuing oral antiviral therapy in a patient with E-antigen negative chronic HBV.

suppressed to as low a level as possible. In addition, if treatment is disconnected, there is a risk of reactivation, which could lead to hepatic decompensation in a patient with cirrhosis. As a result, it is currently recommended that all patients who are HBsAg positive and have cirrhosis remain on antiviral therapy lifelong.

References

1. Tan J, Lok AS. Update on viral hepatitis: 2006. *Curr Opin Gastroenterol.* 2007;23:263-267.
2. Hoofnagle JH, Doo E, Liang TJ, Fleischer R, Lok AS. Management of hepatitis B: summary of a clinical research workshop. *Hepatology.* 2007;45:1056-1075.
3. Keeffe EB, Marcellin P. New and emerging treatment of chronic hepatitis B. *Clin Gastroenterol Hepatol.* 2007;5:285-294.

How Do I Know When a Patient Receiving an Oral Antiviral Agent Has Developed Resistance and What Do I Do When This Happens?

Mitchell L. Shiffman, MD

Resistance is the major limitation when utilizing an oral antiviral agent for the treatment of chronic hepatitis B virus (HBV). Although it is commonly believed that resistant mutations develop in response to treatment with antiviral agents, the great majority of mutations that convey resistance to antiviral therapy are actually preexisting.[1] Mutations are single nucleotide substitutions (SNPs) that occur in the viral genome. This changes the nucleic acid sequence of a viral gene. In many cases these SNPs have no effect on the amino acid sequence, structure, or function of the protein produced by this genetic mutation. However, in some cases an SNP may change a critical amino acid within the protein product of a gene, and this may have a wide range of effects, as listed in Table 12-1. Some mutations are lethal and prevent the virus from reproducing itself. Such mutated viral strains cease to exist soon after they are formed. Some mutations alter proteins so that they are no longer produced or recognized by serologic testing. In patients with chronic HBV the most common example of this is an SNP that prevents the production of E-antigen. Other SNPs in the HBV genome cause changes to the amino acid sequence of S-antigen or core protein, which in some cases may prevent these proteins or their antibodies from being recognized by standard serologic tests utilized to assess for HBV infection (see Question 9). Other SNPs may affect the ability of antiviral agents to suppress HBV replication.

SNPs within the viral genome occur randomly at regular intervals. As a result, most viruses, including HBV, exist as a family of genetically similar but distinct viral species, as illustrated in Figure 12-1. In general, the naturally occurring form of the virus dominates and is present in the highest concentration. This is referred to as the wild type of the virus. Mutated forms of the virus are generally present at much lower concentrations.

Table 12-1

Ways in Which a Single Nucleotide Polymorphism May Affect a Viral Protein

- No effect
- Render the virus nonviable
- Increase or decrease the virulence of the virus
- Reduce the ability of the virus to reproduce
- Alter the conformation of a viral protein so it is no longer recognized by a serologic assay
- Reduce the binding and effectiveness of one or more antiviral agents

---

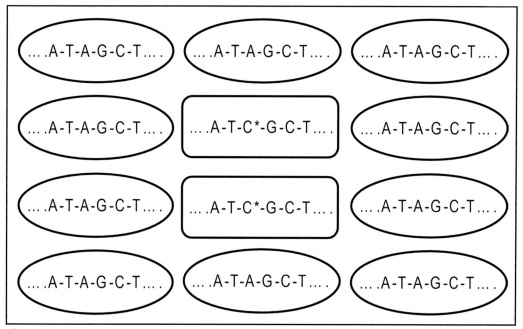

Figure 12-1. Schematic illustrating the concept of how SNPs yield a family of closely related virons. The "wild type" virus appears is covered by an oval envelope and dominates (it is present at much high concentration). The mutated virus has a SNP at position 3 where adenosine has been replaced by cytosine (*). This SNP has caused an amino acid change to a protein of major significance because it has caused a conformational change to the virus envelope (from an oval to a rectangular shape).

In some cases this may be because the mutated vial species is less virulent or replicates at a slower rate than does wild-type virus.

Many SNPs have no significant effect on the virus and/or its protein products, and the mutated species remains sensitive to antiviral agents. Drug-resistant virus emerges when a particular SNP alters an amino acid that is essential for an antiviral agent to bind to and inhibit the action of this protein. When a patient with a drug-resistant viral species is treated with an antiviral agent, there is an initial decline in the serum level of virus because

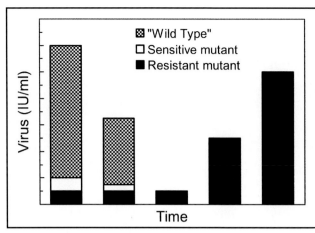

Figure 12-2. Emergence and recognition of viral resistance over time. The total serum level of virus is the sum of "wild type" and mutated species. Both "wild type" and many mutated species are sensitive to antiviral therapy. When anti-viral therapy is initiated those viral species that are sensitive to anti-viral therapy are suppressed. Over time, species that are resistant to the anti-viral agent proliferate cause an increase in serum level of virus and resistance is recognized.

the dominant wild-type virus remains sensitive to the antiviral agent. However, after the concentration of wild-type virus declines to low levels, the resistant species will be able to proliferate more efficiently simply because there is less wild-type virus utilizing the nucleic acid substrate, and as the concentration of resistant virus increases, so does the overall concentration of the total viral pool. This sequence, where wild-type virus is replaced by resistant virus in response to treatment with an antiviral agent, is illustrated in Figure 12-2.

SNPs that convey resistance to each of the antiviral agents currently utilized for treatment of chronic HBV have been well described.[2] A common SNP found in the HBV polymerase gene that conveys resistance to several antiviral agents is the M204I mutation, where methionine is replaced by isoleucine at position 204 within the HBV polymerase. This single amino acid change reduces the ability of lamivudine, telbivudine, and entecovir to bind to the HBV polymerase and reduces the effectiveness of these drugs to inhibit HBV replication. In contrast, this mutation does not affect the ability of adefovir dipivoxil to bind to HBV polymerase and inhibit HBV replication. A separate mutation of the HBV polymerase, N236T, where asparagine is replaced by threonine at position 236, conveys resistance to adefovir but does not affect the effectiveness of either lamivudine, telbivudine, or entecovir. Thus, adefovir can be utilized to treat virus that is resistant to lamivudine, telbivudine, or entecovir; and any of these agents can be utilized to treat virus that is resistant to adefovir. In some cases, multiple or unique mutations of the HBV polymerase may produce a viral species that is resistant to lamivudine and adefovir. Recent studies have suggested that entecovir binds with higher affinity to the HBV polymerase than either lamivudine or telbivudine. Thus, although the M204I mutation may reduce the potency of entecovir, this agent typically remains an effective inhibitor of HBV polymerase unless other mutations are also present.

The frequency at which resistance is observed with the various antiviral agents available for treatment of HBV is summarized in Table 10-2.[3] Unfortunately, SNPs that convey resistance to both lamivudine and telbivudine occur frequently. As a result, 20% to 25% of patients are found to be resistant to these agents within the first year. Over subsequent years, the frequency of lamivudine resistance increases to nearly 70%. Telbivudine has only recently been approved for treatment of chronic HBV and as a result the experience with this agent is limited. However, given that telbivudine has a similar rate of resistance as lamivudine during the first year, resistance would be expected to increase in subse-

Table 12-2

Rates of Virologic Resistance Which Emerge During Treatment With Some of the Currently Available Antiviral Agent

Agent	Resistance Rate
Lamivudine	24% after 1 year
	67% after 5 years
Adefovir Dipivoxil	3% after 2 years
	29% after 5 years
Entecovir	1% after 3 years

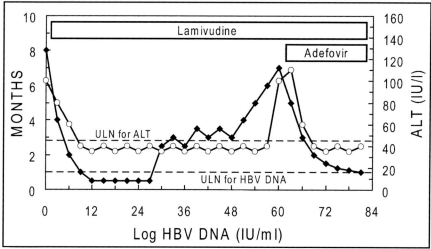

Figure 12-3. Emergence of virologic and clinical resistance in a patient with chronic HBV initially treated with lamivudine. Initially, there is excellent viral suppression in response to lamivudine and this is maintained for over 24 months. Virologic resistance emerges at 30 months but remains at low viral levels for over 1 year before clinical resistance emerges. Ideally, a second anti-viral agent, preferably adefovir dipivoxil, should have been added as serum HBV DNA began to rise at month 52 and before clinical resistance developed at month 60.

quent years with telbivudine as well. Adefovir dipivoxil has a much lower rate of resistance, less than 10% after 3 years. This suggests that the mutation that coneys resistance to adefovir occurs far less frequently in nature than the mutation that coneys resistance to lamivudine or telbivudine. Although entecovir binds to the HBV polymerase active site with much greater affinity than either lamivudine or telbivudine, the presence of mutations that convey resistance to lamivudine should reduce the effectiveness of entecovir and thereby increase the likelihood of resistance to entecovir. Indeed, 18% of patients with lamivudine resistance are also found to be resistant to entecovir within the first year of treatment.

Resistance has been subdivided into 2 categories: virologic and clinical.[3] These patterns are illustrated in Figure 12-3. Virologic resistance is characterized by a recurrence or an increase in the serum level of the virus despite continued use of the antiviral agent. Clinical resistance occurs when viral resistance causes symptoms. In the case of HBV, virologic resistance is recognized when HBV DNA recurs after initially becoming undetectable while being treated with a particular antiviral agent, and clinical resistance occurs when the patient develops hepatitis, an elevation in serum amino transferase (AT) activity. In general, the level of HBV DNA required to cause clinical resistance is approximately 1 million IU/mL. As virologic resistance emerges, many patients may have recurrence of HBV DNA, but at low levels in serum, for many months or years before the serum level of HBV DNA increases significantly and clinical resistance occurs. It remains unclear whether any action, or change in therapy, is required for patients with low levels of virologic resistance. However, recent data suggest that once the serum level of resistant virus exceeds 1 million copies/mL, the effectiveness of an alternative antiviral agent is reduced. Thus, patients with virologic resistance should be monitored closely for progressive elevations in serum HBV DNA. Treatment should be altered if the serum level of HBV DNA increases stepwise over time and before clinical resistance emerges. The question of whether to switch to or add an alternative antiviral agent in a patient who has developed antiviral resistance remains controversial. However, experts currently favor adding a second antiviral agent that acts at a different site of action. Thus, resistance to lamivudine, telbivudine, or entecovir should be treated by adding adefovir, and vice versa. There is no rationale for utilizing either lamivudine, telbivudine, or entecovir simultaneously, since each of these drugs have the same site of action.

Testing for resistant species of HBV has recently become clinically available. Although some experts advocate performing resistance testing at baseline and utilizing this information to select a specific antiviral agent for treatment, the majority of experts see no real advantage to this. The two most commonly utilized antiviral agents for treatment of chronic HBV, adefovir dipivoxil and entecovir, have very low rates of viral resistance and therefore testing all patients for resistance is unlikely to be cost-effective. In addition, performing resistance testing at baseline does not guarantee that a resistant species will not emerge in the future. Identifying the emergence of virologic resistance in a patient receiving antiviral therapy can be ready accomplished by assessing HBV DNA regular intervals as illustrated in Figure 12-3. Performing resistance testing at this point is rarely useful and does not help to select an alternative agent to utilize since the choices are limited.

Over time, multiple mutations of HBV may emerge and the patient may become resistant to several combinations of antiviral agents. Peginterferon may be a useful agent for treatment of chronic HBV in the patient with multiple drug-resistant species regardless of E-antigen status. Since peginterferon acts to suppress virus via indirect mechanisms, including immune modulation, resistance to peginterferon does not occur. The use of peginterferon for treatment of chronic HBV was discussed in Question 10. In the patient who is already resistant to multiple antiviral agents, the strategy and duration of peginterferon therapy may need to be revised. Unfortunately, no clinical trials or other data are currently available to guide such therapy.

In summary, mutations in the HBV genome are the result of SNPs that occur naturally and generally exist prior to instituting treatment with an antiviral agent. Some mutations occur more frequently than others, and this explains the various resistance rates to the antiviral agents utilized to treat chronic HBV. Recognizing virologic resistance is important and requires that HBV DNA be assessed at regular intervals for as long as the patient remains on antiviral therapy. The development of virologic resistance does not immediately require that treatment be altered as long as the patient is closely monitored. However, a second antiviral agent should be added before the patient develops overt clinical resistance.

References

1. Ghany M, Liang TJ. Drug targets and molecular mechanisms of drug resistance in chronic hepatitis B. *Gastroenterology.* 2007;132:1574-1585.
2. Fung SK, Fontana RJ. Management of drug-resistant chronic hepatitis B. *Clin Liver Dis.* 2006;10:275-302.
3. Hadziyannis SJ, Papatheodoridis GV. Hepatitis B e antigen-negative chronic hepatitis B: natural history and treatment. *Semin Liver Dis.* 2006;26:130-141.

How Do I Treat a Patient Who Is Coinfected With Chronic Hepatitis B and C Viruses?

Mitchell L. Shiffman, MD

Both the hepatitis B virus (HBV) and hepatitis C virus (HCV) are transmitted via percutaneous exposure and, as a result, it is not surprising that some patients acquire both viruses either simultaneously or sequentially. In general, HBV is far easier to transmit than HCV. This is because the serum level of HBV is on the order of 10-fold to 100-fold greater than HCV and that HBV is also found in high concentrations in many other body fluids. As a result, HBV can be transmitted vertically from mother to infant and also sexually through intimate contact. In contrast, the concentration of HCV in body fluids is significantly lower than in the bloodstream and, as a result, it is uncommon for HCV to be transmitted vertically or through sexual activity except in the case of human immunodeficiency virus (HIV) coinfection (see Questions 14 and 15). Thus, the vast majority of patients who are coinfected with HCV and HBV acquired these viruses by utilizing intravenous drugs or through other high-risk percutaneous exposures.

Evaluation of Patients With Coinfection

Over 90% of adults exposed to HBV develop acute icteric hepatitis, mount an appropriate immune response, spontaneously resolve this virus, and develop anti-hepatitis B surface (anti-HBs). Those patients who develop chronic HBV remain hepatitis B surface antigen (HbsAg) positive. In contrast, most persons exposed to HCV develop an acute hepatitis without becoming icteric and approximately 80 to 85% develop chronic infection. All individuals exposed to HCV, whether they develop chronic infection or resolve this virus, are anti-HCV positive. When individuals become coinfected with HBV and HCV, 1 of 4 scenarios may occur: they may resolve HBV and develop chronic HCV; they

Table 13-1

Interpretation of Serologic Studies in Patients With HBV and HCV Coinfection

Interpretation	HBV Surface Antigen (+)	Anti-HCV (+)
Active E-antigen positive HBV and HCV	E-antigen (+) anti-E (−) HBV DNA > 10^5 IU/mL	HCV RNA detectable
Active E-antigen negative HBV and HCV	E-antigen (−) Anti-E (+) HBV DNA > 10^5 IU/mL	HCV RNA detectable
Active HBV and inactive HCV	E-antigen (+) or (−) E-antigen (+) or (−) HBV DNA > 10^5 IU/mL	HCV RNA undetectable
Inactive HBV and active HCV	E-antigen (+) or (−) E-antigen (+) or (−) HBV DNA undetectable	HCV RNA detectable
Inactive HBV and HCV	E-antigen (−) anti-E (+) HBV DNA undetectable	HCV RNA undetectable
Inactive HBV, inactive HCV, and active HDV	E-antigen (+) or (−) E-antigen (+) or (−) HBV DNA undetectable Anti-HDV (+) HDV RNA detectable	HCV RNA undetectable

may resolve HCV and develop chronic HBV; they may resolve both viruses; or they may develop chronic infection with both HBV and HCV.[1] These possibilities can be recognized by serologic and virologic testing for these two viruses, as outlined in Table 13-1.

In some cases of HBV and HCV coinfection, one of the two viruses may inhibit the other.[2] This is often because one of the viruses is replicating at a much faster rate and inhibiting the replication of the other. After treatment and eradication of the dominant virus the other virus may then become active. An example of this is provided in Figure 13-1. This patient with E-antigen–negative HBV has high levels of HBV DNA and undetectable HCV RNA at baseline. An oral antiviral agent is initiated for the treatment of HBV, and as the serum level of HBV DNA declines, HCV RNA appears in serum. In some cases, depending upon the treatment utilized (see below), reactivation of the apparently dormant virus may not occur until after the treatment has been discontinued. This is most commonly seen with peginterferon since this agent has activity against both of these viruses. It is therefore important that patients with coinfection be monitored on a regular basis for both viruses during and after treatment, even though one of the viruses may be inactive at the time treatment is initiated.

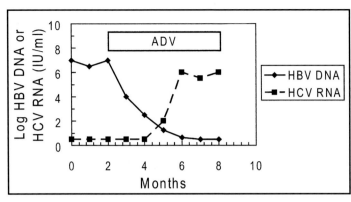

Figure 13-1. HBV DNA and HCV RNA over time in a patient with serologic evidence of both HBV and HCV infection. At baseline the patient was positive for HB surface antigen, anti-HCV and HBV DNA. However, HCV RNA was undetectable. After treatment with adefovir dipivoxil (ADV) was initiated HBV DNA declined. However, when HBV DNA became undetectable HCV RNA began to rise.

Patients with serologic markers for HBV and HCV may have undetectable HBV DNA and HCV RNA and therefore appear to have resolved both of these viral infections. However, another possible explanation for this finding is that these patients have triple infection with hepatitis D virus (HDV). In this setting, the high replication rate of HDV may suppress both HBV and HCV to levels that are undetectable by current virologic assays. As a result, patients with HBV and HCV coinfection should be tested for HDV.[3]

Treatment of Patients With Coinfection

The indications, factors to consider, and need for liver biopsy prior to initiating treatment in a patient with HBV and HCV coinfection are basically the same as in patients with only an HCV or HBV infection, as discussed in Questions 3, 9, and 10. However, the role and need for liver biopsy prior to initiating treatment may be more important in patients with coinfection, particularly when one of the two viruses is inactive or dormant. As noted above, in the setting of coinfection, one virus may inhibit the replication of the other. Thus, if the active virus is not causing significant liver injury, as assessed by liver histology, treatment may actually worsen the situation by causing reactivation of the previously dormant virus. Thus, all patients with HBV and HCV coinfection should be thoroughly evaluated and all of the implications of treatment should be carefully weighed before treatment is initiated.

Patients with E-antigen–positive HBV and HCV coinfection are excellent candidates for treatment with peginterferon alfa-2a since this medication is indicated and approved for both viral infections.[4] Although ribavirin is not useful in the treatment of HBV, this medication significantly enhances the likelihood that the HCV coinfection will be treated successfully. Such patients should therefore be started on standard doses of combination therapy (peinterferon alfa-2a 180 mcg/wk and ribavirin 1000 to 1200 mg/d). There are currently no data to suggest that coinfection alters the response of either of these viruses to peginterferon. Once treatment is initiated, HCV RNA should be monitored at regular intervals as outlined in Question 4. If the patient with HCV genotype 1 fails to achieve an early virologic response, ribavirin should be stopped and peginterferon continued for another 24 weeks to complete the 48-week treatment course recommended for HBV infection. If HCV RNA responds to treatment and becomes undetectable within 24 weeks of treatment, then both peginterferon and ribavirin should be continued for the appropriate duration of therapy based upon the HCV genotype, as discussed in Question 4. Patients should then be monitored at regular intervals for sustained virologic response or relapse in the case of HCV and for seroconversion in the case of HBV. If seroconversion does not occur within 6 months after discontinuing treatment, then the use of an oral antiviral agent to treat HBV can be considered.

Patients with E-antigen–negative HBV and HCV coinfection should also be treated with peginterferon and ribavirin. Although seroconversion does not occur in patients with E-antigen–negative HBV, approximately 33% of these patients do respond to peginterferon, become HBV DNA undetectable, and remain so for many years after this treatment has been completed. If the HBV infection does not respond to peginterferon or reactivates at some time after this treatment is completed, than the use of an oral antiviral agent for treatment of HBV can be considered.

In patients where HBV is either inactive or dormant, the HCV infection can be treated with peginterferon and ribavirin. Patients with active HBV but dormant or resolved HCV can be treated with either peginterferon or an oral antiviral agent. However, with either scenario, both viruses should be monitored on a regular basis during and after treatment to ensure that reactivation of the previously inactive or dormant virus has not occurred. This is especially important in those patients where the active virus has responded to treatment.

References

1. Squadrito G, Orlando ME, Pollicino T, et al. Virological profiles in patients with chronic hepatitis C and overt or occult HBV infection. *Am J Gastroenterol.* 2002;97:1518-1523.
2. Cacciola I, Pollicino T, Squadrito G, Cerenzia G, Orlando ME, Raimondo G. Occult hepatitis B virus infection in patients with chronic hepatitis C liver disease. *N Engl J Med.* 1999;341:22-26.
3. Shukla NB, Poles MA. Hepatitis B virus infection: co-infection with hepatitis C virus, hepatitis D virus, and human immunodeficiency virus. *Clin Liver Dis.* 2004;8:445-460.
4. Urganci N, Gulec S, Dogan S, Nuhoglu A. Interferon and ribavirin treatment results of patients with HBV-HCV co-infection cured of childhood malignancies. *Int J Infect Dis.* 2006;10:453-457.

SECTION III

LIVER DISEASE IN PATIENTS WITH HIV INFECTION

How Does Having HIV Affect the Likelihood That My Patient With Chronic Hepatitis C Will Develop Cirrhosis?

Kevin M. Comar, MD
Richard K. Sterling, MD, MSc, FACP, FACG

Due to overlapping routes of transmission, the seroprevalence of hepatitis C virus (HCV) among human immunodeficiency virus (HIV)-affected individuals is approximately 15% to 30%, which translates to more than 200,000 to 300,000 individuals in the United States alone.[1] The risk of coinfection is directly dependent on the risk factor associated with acquiring the infection. Intravenous drug use (IVDU) or blood product transfusions carry a much higher prevalence rate (80 to 90%) compared to sexual transmission (5 to 10%). The use of highly active antiretroviral therapy (HAART) has decreased the morbidity and mortality of opportunistic infections in HIV, and now liver disease caused by HCV is a leading cause of morbidity and mortality among coinfected patients.[2,3] This sharp increase in the number of deaths due to end-stage liver disease among the HIV–HCV coinfected population has lead to the increased recognition of HCV by HIV providers. Subsequently, this increased recognition has drawn attention to the natural history of HCV in the setting of HIV and the impact of HCV on HIV.

The effect of HIV coinfection on the progression of HCV remains unclear. Graham et al,[4] in a meta-analysis, found that the relative risk for coinfected patients developing histological cirrhosis was 2.07 (95% CI, 1.40 to 3.07) compared to HCV monoinfected patients. However, most of the studies used in the meta-analysis to determine the impact of HIV on HCV included only patients with elevated liver chemistries and/or obvious signs of liver disease. It is important to note that since approximately 30 to 50% of patients with HIV–HCV coinfection have normal alanine aminotransferase (ALT) at the time of biopsy, excluding these patients may have led to an overestimation of HCV disease severity. When we looked at our coinfected population and stratified patients by normal or abnormal ALT, we observed no significant differences in disease severity, as assessed by the Knodell hepatic activity index (HAI), in its inflammation or fibrosis components.[5] In fact, the prevalence of advanced fibrosis (bridging fibrosis or cirrhosis) in those with normal ALT was 26%, which highlights the importance of liver biopsy in this subset of coinfected individuals.

When compared to those with HCV alone, a retrospective cohort study conducted among HCV-infected veterans controlling for demographics (age, race, and gender) and other comorbidities (toxic hepatitis, chronic HBV, diabetes, coagulation disorder, drug dependence, and alcoholism) found that HCV–HIV coinfection was not a significant predictor of cirrhosis (HR = 0.99, 95% CI: 0.87 to 1.12, p = 0.83).[6] However, age, Hispanic ethnicity, toxic hepatitis, chronic HBV, diabetes, coagulation disorder, and alcoholism were significant positive predictors in the model, regardless of HIV status. The model restricted to the HAART era (post-1995) showed similar findings to that of the entire cohort model; however, in the model restricted to the pre-HAART era, HCV-HIV coinfection was a significant predictor for cirrhosis (HR = 1.48, 95% CI: 1.06 to 2.07, p = 0.02). Other variables that had a significant positive association with cirrhosis in the pre-HAART era model were age, toxic hepatitis, chronic HBV, diabetes, and coagulation disorder.

When evaluating the effects of HIV coinfection on the progression to liver disease, one must also consider the specific effect of HAART on HCV.[7] HAART therapy is an essential component in the management of HIV-infected patients. The increased risk of drug-induced hepatotoxicity in patients with concomitant HCV infection has been well documented and, as a consequence, coinfected patients are more likely to require the discontinuation of HAART. Although most reports have focused on severe elevations in liver enzymes (grade 3: 5 to 10× upper limit normal [ULN] and grade 4: ≥10× ULN), more mild to moderate (>1.25 to 5× ULN) elevations are also frequently seen in patients on HAART. The proposed mechanisms for each class of antiretroviral agents are shown in Table 14-1. In coinfected patients fortunate enough not to develop hepatotoxicity, the impact of HAART regimens as a whole on HCV-related liver disease is controversial. In a retrospective analysis, Benhamou and colleagues[2] observed that protease inhibitor (PI) therapy may not accelerate progression to HCV-related cirrhosis.[8] In addition, the chronic use of antiretroviral therapy utilizing PIs, reduction of alcohol consumption, and maintenance of a high CD4 count had a beneficial impact on liver fibrosis progression in HIV–HCV coinfected patients. On the contrary, a recent study of our patients was unable to detect any significant differences in the spectrum of liver disease in patients whose HAART regimen contained a PI compared to those who did not.[9] It is believed the discordant results may have been due to the populations studied, patient demographics, alcohol use, and the dynamic changes that have occurred in anti-HIV therapy. For instance, in the Benhamou study,[2] use of nonnucleoside reverse transcriptase inhibitors (NNRTIs) in a PI treatment group were not given and of those 119 patients not taking a PI, 76 (66%) were on NRTIs alone, 40 (33%) were on no antiretroviral medications, and only 3 patients were taking both nucleoside reverse transcriptase inhibitor (NRTIs) and NNRTIs. Furthermore, patients on a PI had a lower CD4 count compared to patients not on a PI (mean 286 vs. 399 cell/mm³; p = 0.001). Therefore, it is unclear whether it is the use of PIs themselves or the lower CD4 count that accounted for less histologic damage observed. In a retrospective analysis of 690 coinfected patients enrolled in APRICOT, a trial in treating HCV in those with

Table 14-1

Hepatotoxicity and HAART*

Class	Mechanism	Manifestation
NRTI	Decrease mitochondrial DNA polymerase gamma	Lactic acidosis, steatosis
NNRTI	Immune hypersensitivity	Lactic acidosis, steatosis, eosinophilic hepatic injury
PI	Inhibit retinoic acid binding protein? Direct cytopathic (RTV) Decrease UDP-glucuronide transfer (IDV, ATV)	Hepatocellular injury Steatosis Increased unconjugated bilirubin
HAART	Immune constitution?	Hepatocellular injury

*NRTI indicates nucleoside reverse transcriptase inhibitor; NNRTI, nonnucleoside reverse transcriptase inhibitor; PI, protease inhibitor; RTV, ritonovir; IDV, indinovir; ATV, atazanavir.

HIV, no significant differences in the proportion with severe fibrosis (approximately 25%) were observed between those on a NNRTI, a PI, or both.[10] Therefore, it is difficult to conclude whether specific PI or NNRTI use is associated with obvious histological benefit or obvious histological worsening of HCV disease.

In conclusion, with advances in HIV treatment, the life expectancy of HIV-infected individuals has been prolonged. As such, liver disease has become a significant cause of morbidity and mortality in those with HCV coinfection. Although studies early on suggested accelerated fibrosis progression, more recent work in the HAART era have shown a similar spectrum of disease in coinfected patients compared to patients with HCV alone. It is clear that ongoing alcohol use is associated with HCV disease progression. Currently, there are no data to support the use of one particular class of HAART and therefore the choice of which drug to use should depend on controlling HIV rather than the potential impact on HCV disease progression. However, because the natural history of HCV in the current HAART era remains unclear, prospective studies using paried biopsies are still needed.

References

1. Sherman KE, Rouster SD, Chung RT, Rajicic N. Hepatitis C Virus prevalence among patients infected with Human Immunodeficiency Virus: a cross-sectional analysis of the US adult AIDS Clinical Trials Group. *Clin Infect Dis*. 2002;34:831-837.
2. Bica I, McGovern B, Dhar R, et al. Increasing mortality due to end-stage liver disease in patients with human immunodeficiency virus infection. *Clin Infect Dis*. 2001;32: 492-497.
3. Darby SC, Ewart DW, Giangrande PL, et al. Mortality from liver cancer and liver disease in haemophilic men and boys in UK given blood products contaminated with hepatitis C. UK Haemophilia Centre Directors' Organisation. *Lancet*. 1997;350:1425-1431.

4. Graham CS, Baden LR, Yu E, et al. Influence of human immunodeficiency virus infection on the course of hepatitis C virus infection: a meta-analysis. *Clin Infect Dis*. 2001;33:562-569.
5. Sterling RK, Contos MJ, Sanyal AJ, et al. The clinical spectrum of hepatitis C virus in HIV coinfection. *J Acquir Immune Defic Syndr*. 2003;32:30-37.
6. Kramer JR, Giordano TP, Souchek J, et al. The effect of HIV coinfection on the risk of cirrhosis and hepatocellular carcinoma in U.S. veterans with hepatitis C. *Am J Gastroenterol*. 2005;100:56-63.
7. Mehta SH, Thomas DL, Torbenson M, et al. The effect of antiretroviral therapy on liver disease among adults with HIV and hepatitis C coinfection. *Hepatology*. 2005;41:123-131.
8. Benhamou Y, Di MV, Bochet M, et al. Factors affecting liver fibrosis in human immunodeficiency virus-and hepatitis C virus-coinfected patients: impact of protease inhibitor therapy. *Hepatology*. 2001;34:283-287.
9. Sterling RK, Wilson MS, Sanyal AJ, et al. Impact of highly active antiretroviral therapy on the spectrum of liver disease in HCV-HIV coinfection. *Clin Gastroenterol Hepatol*. 2004;2:432-439.
10. Sterling RK, Lissen E, Clumeck N, et al. Effects of protease inhibitors and non-nucleoside reverse transcriptase inhibitors on liver histology in HIV/HCV co-infection. Analysis of patients enrolled in the AIDS Pegasys Ribavirin International Co-Infection Trial (APRICOT). 2006. Boston, MA, 12th Conference on Retroviruses and Opportunistic Infections (CROI). Abstract 951.

WHICH PATIENTS WITH CHRONIC HEPATITIS C AND HIV COINFECTION SHOULD BE TREATED WITH PEGINTERFERON AND RIBAVIRIN?

Kevin M. Comar, MD
Richard K. Sterling, MD, MSc, FACP, FACG

Once a coinfected individual is identified, an evaluation should be made by a multidisciplinary team to determine whether the patient is a candidate for anti-HCV treatment. Highly active antiretroviral therapy (HAART) in coinfected patients should follow the current recommendations for initiation of antiviral human immunodeficiency virus (HIV) monoinfected therapy with a few exceptions as outlined in the following text. The goals of hepatitis C virus (HCV) therapy in the setting of HIV mirror those of treatment in the HCV monoinfected patient, including virologic eradication and histological improvement with prevention of progression to cirrhosis. As in the setting of the monoinfected HCV patient, the current optimal regimen is with pegylated interferon and ribavirin. A simple algorithm for treating HCV in those coinfected is provided in Figure 15-1.

Patients in which HCV therapy is about to be initiated and who have CD4 counts close to the threshold for initiation of HAART should be considered for pre-emptive therapy HIV, secondary to risk of decrease in CD4 cell count during IFN-based anti-HCV therapy. As with the HCV-monoinfected patient, anti-HCV therapy in the coinfected patient should be avoided in those with previous or current liver decompensation, a history of severe neuropsychiatric disorders, or in patients with current heavy alcohol or illegal drug use. In patients who are not candidates for HCV therapy secondary to neurophychiatric disorders or active drug abuse, professional psychiatric management and detoxification programs are recommended with the possibility of treatment in the future.

When determining whether a coinfected patient is a candidate for anti-HCV therapy, careful attention should be given to CD4 counts, as the response to anti-HCV therapy may be dependent on CD4 cell count. Moreover, patients with CD4 counts below

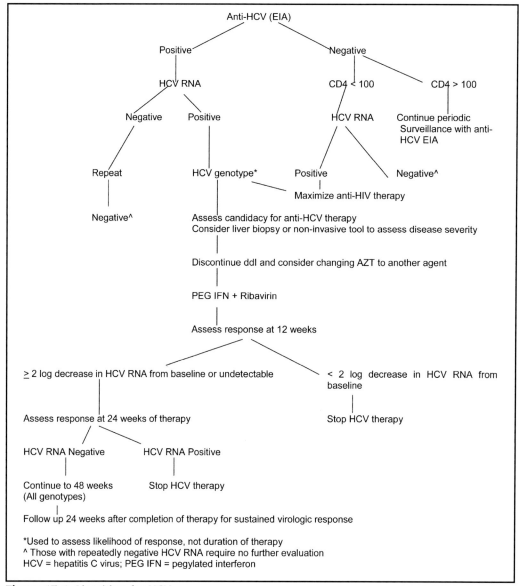

Figure 15-1. Algorithm for HCV.

100 are at higher risk for opportunistic infections after initiation of anti HCV therapy. Preferably, anti-HCV therapy candidates should have a CD4 count above 200 cells/μL. In individuals with CD4 count of less than 200 cells/μL, therapy should be avoided unless they have undetectable HIV RNA. In those with low counts (<200) and detectable HIV RNA levels, initiation of antiretroviral therapy is suggested as well as prophylactic therapy for opportunistic infections. Ideally, these patients may increase their CD4 counts to the point where they can become candidates for anti-HCV therapy. The decision to begin anti-HCV therapy should be determined after careful consideration of factors such as the severity of liver disease and classic predictors of response to anti-HCV therapy (HCV genotype, viral load, age, BMI).

Patients with normal serum aminotransferases should still be considered for treatment if the histology indicates a significant degree of inflammation or fibrosis. Traditionally, liver biopsy has been used as a key diagnostic tool in the patient with HCV. However, the role of liver biopsy for treatment decision purposes in coinfection remains controversial.[1] As with any invasive procedure, there are significant risks including bleeding, pain, perforation of bowel or lung, sampling error, financial cost of the procedure, and anxiety to both patient and physician. We believe that liver biopsy is important as it remains the "gold standard" in assessing liver disease severity and prognosis and provides information regarding the presence of HAART hepatotoxicity or other comorbid conditions such as hepatic steatosis. Also, knowing the severity of liver disease helps in determining how hard to push HCV therapy in those who are not tolerating it well. However, because of the potential risks, several noninvasive models to assess disease severity have been developed, such as the FIB-4 index.[2]

Current recommendations are based on recent trials that have evaluated their use (Table 15-1). The APRICOT study[3] and the ACTG A5071 study[4] both compared PEG-IFN alfa-2a plus ribavirin to standard IFN plus ribavirin. The APRICOT study included an arm to evaluate PEG-IFN monotherapy. Results from this study demonstrated a significantly higher sustained virologic response rated (SVR, defined as HCV RNA <50 IU/mL 24 weeks following treatment for 48 weeks) among all genotypes for those patients receiving PEG-IFN plus RVN versus those receiving standard IFN combination therapy (40% vs. 12%; odds ratio, 5.40; 95% confidence interval [CI], 3.20 to 9.12; $p < .001$) and versus those receiving PEG-IFN monotherapy (40% vs. 20%; odds ratio 2.89; 95% CI 1.83 to 4.58; $p < 0.001$). As seen in the HCV monoinfected population, higher SVRs were achieved with HCV genotype 2 or 3 compared to genotype 1 in all three treatment arms. In addition, patients with HCV genotype 1 with high HCV RNA levels (>800,000 IU/mL) had lower response rates in all three treatment arms compared to those with low HCV RNA levels (<800,000 IU/mL).[3] Similar results were seen in the ACTG A5071 study, a two-armed study that used a stepwise dosing of RVN in the PEG-IFN combination arm as well as a dose reduction from 6 MIU to 3 MIU in the standard IFN arm. Significantly higher SVR was seen with patients receiving PEG-IFN compared to standard IFN (18% vs. 8%, $p = 0.03$), with only 14% of genotype 1 patients achieving SVR with PEG-IFN compared to 73% of patients with genotype 2 or 3 ($p < 0.001$). Interestingly, a detectable HIV RNA level at entry into the study was found to be a predictor of SVR in multivariate analysis (OR 3.55, 95% CI 1.19 to 10.6; $p = 0.023$).[4] Both the RIBAVIC study[5] and the Spanish study by Laguno et al[6] evaluated combination therapy with PEG-IFN alfa-2b and RVN compared to the combination therapy using standard IFN. In general, both the French[5] and Spanish[6] groups demonstrated significantly higher SVR in all patients treated with PEG-IFN compared to standard interferon including those with genotypes 2 and 3.

Similar to monoinfection trials, the predictive value of early virologic response (EVR, defined as a 2 log or more decrease in the HCV RNA level by week 12) have been confirmed in managing HCV in HIV coinfection. In the APRICOT study, 71% of patients demonstrated an EVR, of whom 56% went on to have an SVR.[3] Of the 29% of patients who had no early virologic response, only 2% went on to have an SVR, none of whom were in the PEG-IFN monotherapy arm or standard IFN arm. Similarly, a negative predictive value of no EVR was 100% in the ACTG A5071 trial.[4] Lastly, because of increased relapse rates in coinfected individuals with only 24 weeks of treatment, those with genotypes 2 and 3 who respond to therapy should receive 48 weeks.

Table 15-1

Clinical Trials With Peg-IFN and Ribavirin in HIV-HCV Coinfection

	APRICOT	RIBAVIC	ACTG A5071	Laguno	Perez-Olmeda
Total cohort/ Peg-IFN + RVN arm	868/289	412/205	133/66	95/52	68
Treatment	Peg-IFN alpha 2a 180 mcg weekly + RVN 800 mg daily	Peg-IFN alpha 2b 1.5 mcg/ kg weekly + RVN 800 mg daily	Peg-IFN alpha 2a 180 mcg weekly + RVN on escalating dose weekly to 1000 mg daily	Peg-IFN alpha 2b 100-150 mcg weekly + RVN 800-1200 mg daily	Peg-IFN alpha 2b 150 mcg weekly for first 12 weeks then 100 mcg weekly + RVN 800 mg daily
Dropout, %	25	39	12	23	21
Age	40	40	45	40	39
% Genotype 1	61	49	77	55	57
Fibrosis score 5 or 6, %	13	16	11	NA	17
HAART, %	85	83	85	94	74
Mean/median CD4 count	520 (Mean)	477 (Median)	495 (Median)	570 (Mean)	591 (Mean)
% Undetectable HIV RNA at baseline	60	70	61	70	76
SVR (overall), %	40				
SVR genotype 1, %	29	17	14	38	24
SVR genotype 2, 3, %	62	44	73 (non-geno-type 1)	53	52

Adverse effects from interferon-based therapy include neutropenia, thrombocytopenia, anemia, influenza-like syndrome, and psychiatric disturbances. Neutropenia and anemia secondary to marrow suppression is often found in HIV patients. Thus, many coinfected patients may benefit from using growth factors including erythropoietin and granulocyte colony stimulating factor during anti-HCV therapy. It is also important to note that hepatic decompensation and liver-related deaths have been documented in coinfected patients who began treatment with mild hepatic decompensation. The spectrum of side effects of anti-HCV therapy, superimposed on the myriad number of side effects from antiretroviral therapy medications, can be taxing for any patient. Higher withdrawal rate due to adverse affects is predictable. Generally, HCV therapy can be used safely in coinfected patients with well-compensated HCV. However, because drug interactions with didanosine (ddI) can lead to increased risk of mitochondrial toxicity, didanosine should not be used in patients receiving ribavirin and ddI should be discontinued for several months prior to the initiation of ribavirin. In the setting of HCV treatment, these mitochondrial toxicities are manifested by pancreatitis and hyperlactatemia. In addition, use of zidovudine (AZT) may exacerbate the anemia associated with ribavirin. Therefore, it is recommended that these drugs not be used during HCV therapy. As in treatment of HCV monoinfection, the development of common adverse effects should not incite an immediate abortion of therapy. Rather, various supportive measures can be initiated, such as epoetin in the case of anemia and antidepressants for symptoms of depression. In attempting to achieve virologic clearance, optimizing the dose of medication and maintaining duration of therapy are critical.[7]

References

1. Sterling RK. Role of liver biopsy in the evaluation of hepatitis C virus in HIV coinfection. *Clin Infect Dis*. 2005; 40(Suppl 5):S270-275.
2. Sterling RK, Lissen E, Clumeck N, et al. Development of a simple noninvasive index to predict significant fibrosis in patients with HIV/HCV coinfection. *Hepatology*. 2006;43:1317-1325.
3. Torriani FJ, Rodriguez-Torres M, Rockstroh JK, et al. Peginterferon Alfa-2a plus ribavirin for chronic hepatitis C virus infection in HIV-infected patients. *N Engl J Med*. 2004;351:438-450.
4. Chung RT, Andersen J, Volberding P, et al. Peginterferon Alfa-2a plus ribavirin versus interferon alfa-2a plus ribavirin for chronic hepatitis C in HIV-coinfected persons. *N Engl J Med*. 2004;351:451-459.
5. Carrat F, Bani-Sadr F, Pol S, et al. Pegylated interferon alfa-2b vs standard interferon alfa-2b, plus ribavirin, for chronic hepatitis C in HIV-infected patients: a randomized controlled trial. *JAMA*. 2004;292:2839-2848.
6. Laguno M, Murillas J, Blanco JL, et al. Peginterferon alfa-2b plus ribavirin compared with interferon alfa-2b plus ribavirin for treatment of HIV/HCV co-infected patients. *AIDS*. 2004;18:F27-F36.
7. Soriano V, Puoti M, Sulkowski M, et al. Care of patients with hepatitis C and HIV co-infection. *AIDS*. 2004; 18: 1-12.

16

Is There a Simple Way to Treat a Patient Who Is Coinfected With Hepatitis B Virus and HIV?

Richard K. Sterling, MD, MSc, FACP, FACG

The simple answer to this question is yes and no. The majority of those infected with human immunodeficiency virus (HIV) have been exposed to hepatitis B virus (HBV). Before you think about initiating anti-HBV therapy, you need to understand the epidemiology and natural history of HBV in those with HIV. Only then can you consider the treatment options.

Epidemiology

Similar to coinfection of HIV and HCV, with shared modes of transmission, there is also concern over the liver-related health risks of HBV-HIV, which were previously overshadowed by the morbidity and mortality of HIV until the introduction of highly active antiretroviral therapy (HAART). It is known that 70% to 90% of patients with HIV show evidence of prior exposure to HBV. In a cohort of 232 HIV-infected patients, 9% suffered from chronic HBV infection (HBsAg positive), 82% of whom had detectable HBeAg and 86% of whom had detectable HBV DNA.[1] This study also showed that coinfection was associated with reduced survival compared to controls.

Natural History

Impact of HIV on HBV

It is now known that the natural history of HBV is altered by the presence of concurrent HIV infection. HIV infection impairs cell-mediated immunity and is likely to modify the course of HBV via uncontrolled viral replication and decreased hepatocellular necrosis. Colin et al[2] investigated the influence of HIV on chronic HBV utilizing biochemical tests and histologic severity indices in a cohort of homosexual non-drug-addicted men, all with HBV with and without HIV. The HIV-HBV–positive patients had lower serum alanine aminotransferase (ALT) levels, lower serum albumin, and higher serum HBV DNA levels compared to those with only HBV. Multivariate analysis also demonstrated that HIV positivity was associated with an increased risk of cirrhosis (relative risk of 4.20) without increased necroinflammatory process. This contrasts somewhat with the findings of an earlier study by Housset et al,[3] who found no difference in mean ALT values, histologic activity index, or prevalence of cirrhosis in HIV-positive versus HIV-negative patients with chronic HBV; however, follow-up analysis in this series found a lower clearance rate of HBV DNA in HIV-positive patients, indicating the impact of coinfection.

The Multicenter Cohort Study (MACS) results demonstrated that coinfected individuals had a higher liver-related mortality rate than those with either HIV or HBV infection alone.[4] Coinfected men were 8 times more likely to die from liver disease than those with HIV alone and were 19 times more likely to die than those with HBV alone. The rate of liver-related death also increased when nadir CD4 count dropped to less than 100, with HBsAg positivity carrying a relative risk of 11.6 with a CD4 count less than 100 compared to a relative risk of 6.8 when cell count was greater than 250. This suggests that identification and comprehensive management of coinfection is paramount to treatment success, especially in the HAART era.

IMPACT OF HBV ON HIV

Little is known about the effect of HBV on HIV, and the idea that HBV could accelerate HIV progression is controversial. HBV is considered predominately hepatotropic but is also lymphotropic. Proteins encoded by the HBV genome may have an effect on HIV replication through the fourth major coding region of the HBV genome, denoted X. The HBV X protein presumably interacts with NF-kB transcription factors to allow the factors to bind to specific HIV long terminal repeat sequences and increases the rate of transcription, thereby enhancing HIV replication in cells coinfected with HIV and HBV. The duration of latency of HIV may also be shortened by the presence of HBV in HIV-infected mononuclear cells that would diminish the antiviral effects of interferons on the replication of HIV.

EVALUATION AND TREATMENT OF HBV IN THE SETTING OF HIV

Chronic HBV effectively behaves as an opportunistic infection in the setting of concurrent HIV infection. All patients found to have HBV should also be tested for HDV and have periodic surveillance for hepatocellular carcinoma (HCC). The determination also needs to be made as to which virus needs treatment—HBV, HIV, or both. All patients with evidence of active HBV infection (HBsAg positive) with HBeAg positive or HBV DNA ≥10^4 copies/mL or 2000 IU/L, evidence of necroinflammation as demonstrated by liver biopsy or elevated ALT, *or* evidence of cirrhosis with HBV DNA ≥10^3 copies/mL (or greater than 200 IU/L) should be considered candidates for treatment. As with the treatment of HBV in patients without coinfection, the necessity of treatment compliance is also a pertinent issue.

Table 16-1

Treatment Options and Antiviral Activity for HBV-HIV Coinfection

Drug	Anti-HBV	Anti-HIV
Interferon	Yes	No
Lamivudine	Yes	Yes
Tenofovir	Yes	Yes
Emtricitabine	Yes	Yes
Adefovir	Yes	No
Entecavir	Yes	No
Telbuvudine	Yes	No

Overall goals in the treatment of chronic HBV are to reduce liver-related mortality, to improve necroinflammation, and to suppress active HBV replication by either significant reduction or clearance of HBV DNA. Treatment should also focus on conversion from active to nonreplicative virus, as reflected by conversion of HBeAg positive to HBeAb positive, and to pursue the disappearance of chronic carrier status. There are also goals unique to those patients with HIV, including the reduction of antiretroviral drug hepatotoxicity and avoidance of any HBV therapy that would negatively impact the patients HIV therapy. The choice of therapy needs to take into account the overall effectiveness, the risk of resistant mutations, and the potential interactions HBV medication will have on HIV therapy. The options for treating HBV and their impact on HIV are outlined in Table 16-1.

Interferon (IFN)

There are little data on the effectiveness of interferon-alpha for the treatment of chronic HBV in the coinfected patient. DiMartino and colleagues[5] performed a retrospective analysis of the influence of coinfection on response to IFN-alpha therapy, virologic status, and progression to cirrhosis in 141 HBeAg positive patients, 69 of whom were also HIV positive. There was no significant short-term response difference to interferon therapy between HIV-positive and HIV-negative patients, but response was poorer in patients with low CD4 count ($<200/mm^3$). However, long-term seroconversion was only 15.4% in coinfected patients compared to 52% in HIV-negative patients. HIV coinfection was also associated with increased frequency of HBV reactivations, 35.7% in HIV-positive versus 9% in HIV-negative patients. The risk of cirrhosis was also increased in coinfected patients with a CD4 count <200 (relative risk 4.57), but IFN-alpha therapy decreased the incidence of HBV cirrhosis regardless of serologic response or HIV status. Although there is little information regarding the use of peginterferon in the HAART era, it may be a viable option is those without cirrhosis.

Lamivudine (LMV)

LMV is a nucleoside analogue that is effective against both HIV and HBV. Fang and colleagues[6] studied the use of HAART containing LMV with comparison of HBV dynamics between HBeAg-positive and HBeAg-negative coinfected patients. Their findings were that the regimen containing LMV effectively suppressed HBV DNA levels by 10^{-3} to 10^{-5}-fold over baseline in coinfected patients, but there was a residual HBV viremia in most HBeAg-positive patients. This suggests that more potent antiviral regimens are needed in HBeAg-positive patients to effectively suppress HBV replication. Also, since the regimen containing LMV did not effectively suppress HBV replication in these patients, regimens containing LMV as a monotherapy for chronic HBV should not be prescribed in coinfected patients with HBeAg positivity without evidence of active hepatitis, due to the high risk of development of HBV resistance to LMV. Benhamou and colleagues[7] detailed this development of LMV resistance in coinfected patients in a study that demonstrated that LMV therapy led to HBV replication inhibition in 86.4% of coinfected patients. However, they also found that there is development of HBV resistance in the YMDD motif of the DNA polymerase to LMV in up to 50% of patients within the first 2 years of treatment, with a roughly linear annual incidence rate of 20% and an expected actuarial survival curve that showed a potential for 91% HBV resistance at 4 years. This pattern of resistance was only observed in HBeAg carriers, but it was also noted that 1 in 9 patients who had seroconverted also developed LMV resistance.

Adefovir (ADV)

ADV is a nucleotide analogue approved for the treatment of chronic hepatitis B. In one large randomized controlled trial of HBeAg-positive patients where 10 mg of ADV was compared to placebo, there was a significant reduction in HBV DNA levels, 3.52 $\log_{10}$ copies/mL with ADV.[8] There was also found to be a biochemical improvement in 55% of patients as well as a 48% rate of histological improvement. However, HBeAg seroconversion was relatively low and occurred in only 14% of patients.

ADV is also effective in those with HBV DNA–positive, HBeAg-negative HBV and in those with LMV resistance. It is important to note that there can be transient elevation of ALT with the initiation of ADV therapy in the coinfected patient, and that ADV at 10 mg/d is not effective against HIV.

Tenofovir (TNF)

TNF is a nucleotide analogue that has activity against both HBV and HIV. Dore and colleagues[9] concluded that TNF had efficacy against HBV in both HAART-experienced and HAART-naïve coinfected patients. There was a mean reduction in HBV DNA by 4 to 5 $\log_{10}$ copies/mL in HAART-experienced patients after 48 weeks of treatment with TNF and a similar reduction in HBV DNA in HAART-naïve patients who received combination therapy with LMV and TNF as a component of initial HAART 3-drug regimen. There was a trend toward reduced YMDD resistance and greater HBV DNA suppression in coinfected patients receiving LMV and TNF as opposed to LMV alone. Nelson and colleagues[10] also studied TNF in a cohort of 20 coinfected patients, 15 of whom had LMV experience. Patients were given TNF in addition to or as part of antiretroviral therapy. They found a significant decrease in HBV DNA and ALT levels and 25% of patients underwent HBeAg seroconversion. It was also concluded that TNF appears to overcome LMV resistance with a 4 $\log_{10}$ reduction in HBV viral load in the study population. Benhamou and colleagues[11] demonstrated the efficacy of TNF against wild-type, presumed precore mutants and LAM-resistant HBV when used as part of HAART in coinfected patients. They used TNF in combination with LMV in both HBeAg-positive and HBeAg-negative patients and found a significant reduction of HBV DNA in both groups, and HBV DNA became undetectable in 29.6% and 81.6% of HBeAg positive and negative patients, respectively. Finally, a recent study by Peters and colleagues[12] on the ACTG A5127 reported similar response of TNF and ADV in a cohort of 52 HIV-HBV coinfected patients.

Emtricitabine (FTC)

FTC is a nucleoside analogue that is similar to LMV and is approved for HIV treatment. It has been shown to produce up to a 3.3 $\log_{10}$ copies/mL serum HBV DNA reduction in coinfected patients but also has been found to have an incidence of 12% of YMDD mutations in patients following 1 year of FTC therapy.[13] However, FTC will have little impact when used alone or in combination with TNF in LMV-experienced patients.

TNF/FTC Combination

Combination of TNF and FTC (Truvada, Gilead Sciences) has become a first-line agent in treating HIV. Because of the potent antiviral effect on HBV, it has become the ideal choice in those needing both HIV and HBV therapy.[14-16] However, its long-term efficacy on HBV DNA suppression is not known and, therefore, those on therapy will require monitoring for emergence of HBV mutations.

Entecavir (ENT)

ENT is a purine-derived nucleoside analogue that is effective against HBV. It has been shown to be very potent against HBV in monoinfected patients, with a 7 $\log_{10}$ copies/mL reduction in HBV DNA and no resistance at 48 weeks in LMV naïve patients, and has shown a mean reduction of HBV DNA by 3.66 $\log_{10}$ copies/mL versus placebo in LMV-resistant coinfected patients. Although effective against LMV-resistant HBV, efficacy is reduced and higher doses are required. However, the recent observation of increases in HIV RNA when used alone in HIV-HBV coinfected patients may limit its use as monotherapy.

Telbivudine

I am not aware of any data on the use of telbivudine in those coinfected with HIV and therefore cannot recommend it as a treatment option at this time.

SUMMARY OF MANAGEMENT OF HIV-HBV COINFECTION

As with hepatitis C virus (HCV), the recognition that HBV is a significant cause of morbidity and mortality in the HIV-infected population has led to significant advances in our understanding of the impact of HIV on HBV disease progression. All patients with evidence of active HBV replication or evidence of necroinflammation should be considered as candidates for treatment, but the optimal time for the initiation of HBV therapy or the

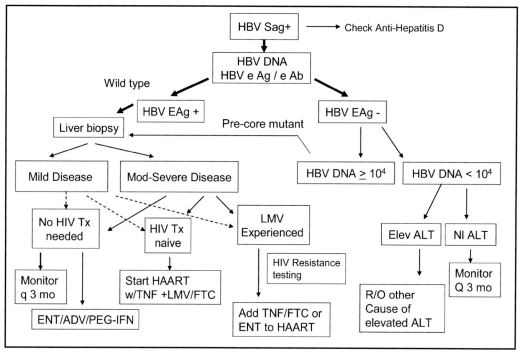

Figure 16-1. Algorithm HBV-HIV infection.

ideal medication regimen is not yet clearly elucidated. Goals of HBV therapy are the loss of active replication, the improvement of necroinflammation, the reduction of liver-related mortality, as well as the reduction of antiretroviral hepatotoxicity. Initial evaluation of the HBsAg-positive patient involves testing HBV DNA viral load, ALT, HBeAg, and HBeAb and excluding coexisting HCV or hepatitis D virus (HDV), as well as screening for HCC. Liver biopsy is also indicated in tandem with immunologic testing to evaluate the degree of necroinflammation and histologic severity of disease. We have outlined a proposed algorithm for the evaluation and management of HBV-HIV coinfection (Figure 16-1). The key is to determine which viruses need treatment. The algorithm starts with determining HBV surface antigen (SAg) status and, if positive, evaluating for HDV coinfection. For those with positive SAg, the next step involves determining HBV DNA level and e-antigen/antibody (eAg/eAb) status. For those with negative eAg, low (<10^4 IU/mL) HBV DNA, and normal (Nl) ALT, no additional HBV therapy is indicated and patients should be monitored every 3 months for reactivation. If HIV requires therapy, then I would avoid LMV and FTC unless TNF is part of HAART. If ALT is elevated (elev), then other causes of hepatitis need to be excluded, such as HCV, HDV, steatohepatitis, alcohol, and medication. If HBV DNA is high (>10^4 IU/mL), then a precore/core mutation is suspected and patients similarly follow those with wild-type eAg-positive HBV and should undergo liver biopsy to assess disease severity. If mild disease is found on biopsy and HIV does not require therapy, these individuals should be monitored for disease flares. For those with moderate to severe disease noted on biopsy, treatment will depend on past or current HIV therapy. If the patient is treatment naïve and does not require HIV therapy, then options include ADV or pegylated interferon (PEG-IFN). If HIV treatment naïve and

HIV also requires treatment, then HAART should include TNF with either FTC or LMV. If LMV experienced, then consider HIV resistance testing and adding TNF with or without LVM or FTC or adding ENT to existing HAART. As with HCV-HIV coinfection, there have been significant advances in the care of HIV patients coinfected with HCV and HBV, giving optimism for this challenging patient population.

References

1. Ockenga J, Tillman HL, Trautwein C, et al. Hepatitis B and C in HIV-infected patients. *J Hepatol.* 1997;27:18-24.
2. Colin JF, Cazals-Hatem D, Loriot MA, et al. Influence of human immunodeficiency virus infection on chronic hepatitis B in homosexual men. *Hepatology.* 1999;29:1306-1310.
3. Housset C, Pol S, Carnot F, et al. Interactions between human immunodeficiency virus-1, hepatitis delta virus and hepatitis B virus infections in 260 chronic carriers of hepatitis B virus. *Hepatology.* 1992;15:578-583.
4. Thio CL, Seaberg EC, Skolasky R, et al. HIV-1, hepatitis B virus, and the risk of liver-related mortality in the Multicenter Cohort Study (MACS). *Lancet.* 2002;360:1921-1926.
5. DiMartino, V, Thevenot T, Colin, JF et al: Influence of HIV infection on the response to interferon therapy and the long-term outcome of chronic hepatitis B. *Gastroenterology.* 2002;123:1812-1822.
6. Fang CT, Chen PJ, Chen MY, et al. Dynamics of plasma hepatitis B virus levels after highly active antiretroviral therapy in patients with HIV infection. *J Hepatol.* 2003;39(6):1028-1035.
7. Benhamou Y, Bochet M, Thibault V, et al. Long-term incidence of hepatitis B virus resistance to lamivudine in human immunodeficiency virus-infected patients. *Hepatology.* 1999;30:1302-1306.
8. Marcellin P, Chang TT, Lim SG, et al. Adefovir dipivoxil for the treatment of hepatitis B e antigen-positive chronic hepatitis B. *N Engl J Med.* 2003;348:808-816.
9. Dore GJ, Cooper DA, Pozniak AL, et al. Efficacy of tenofovir disoproxil fumarate in antiretroviral therapy-naive and -experienced patients coinfected with HIV-1 and hepatitis B virus. *J Infect Dis.* 2004;189(7):1185-1192.
10. Nelson M, Portsmouth S, Stebbing J, et al. An open-label study of tenofovir in HIV-1 and Hepatitis B virus co-infected individuals. *AIDS.* 2003;17(1):F7-10.
11. Benhamou Y, Fleury H, Trimoulet P, et al: Anti-hepatitis B virus efficacy of tenofovir disoproxil fumarate in HIV-infected patients. *Hepatology.* 2006;43:548-555.
12. Peters MG, Anderson J, Lynch P, et al. Randomized controlled study of tenofovir and adefovir in chronic hepatitis B virus and HIV infection: ACTG A5127. *Hepatology.* 2006;44:1110-1116.
13. Snow A, Harris J, Borroto-Esoda K, et al: Emtricitabine therapy for hepatitis infection in HIV + patients co-infected with hepatitis B: efficacy and genotypic findings in antiretroviral treatment naïve patients. 11th conference on retroviruses and opportunistic infection. San Francisco, CA;2004. p. 836 [abstract].
14. Thio CL. Hepatitis B virus infection in HIV-infected persons. *Current Hepatitis Reports.* 2004;3:91-97.
15. Nunez M, Puoti M, Camino N, Soriano V. Treatment of chronic hepatitis B in the human immunodeficiency virus-infected patient: present and future. *Clin Infect Dis.* 2003;37:1678-1685.
16. Benhamou Y. Antiretroviral therapy and HIV/hepatitis B coinfection. *Clin Infect Dis.* 2004;38(Suppl2)98-103.
17. Pessoa W, Gazzard B, Huang A, et al. Entecavir in HIV/HBV co-infected patients: safety and efficacy in a phase II study (ETV-038). Conference on retroviruses and opportunistic infections, Boston, MA; 2005. p. 123 [abstract].

WHAT THINGS COULD CAUSE MY PATIENT WITH HIV TO DEVELOP JAUNDICE?

Richard K. Sterling, MD, MSc, FACP, FACG

When evaluating the cause of jaundice in the human immunodeficiency virus (HIV)-positive patient, the first thing to determine is whether the patient is in acute liver failure (ALF) because this is a true emergency that requires hospitalization. If evidence of new-onset coagulopathy or encephalopathy is present, in the absence of preexisting liver disease, patients should be admitted and managed as ALF. Because those with HIV may be at increased risk for acute hepatitis A and B, or superinfection of hepatitis D in those with chronic B, these causes should be at the top of the list in any HIV patient with ALF. In the early days of HIV therapy with nucleoside reverse transcriptase inhibitors (NRTIs) such as zidovudine (AZT), there were several patients who developed severe lactic acidosis associated with steatosis and liver failure. However, with recent advances in HIV therapy, this is now uncommon and patients with HIV and acute liver failure should undergo similar evaluation as those without HIV.

Once ALF has been excluded, the next step is to determine the pattern and chronicity of liver injury. In those with an acute cholestatic pattern (elevations in alkaline phosphatase and gamma-glutamyl transferase, GGT), I would next proceed with liver imaging to determine whether there is mechanical obstruction or bile duct dilatation. If biliary obstruction is present, then consider endoscopic retrograde cholangiopancreatography (ERCP) and proceed as with any other obstructed patient. If there is no evidence of obstruction or bile duct dilatation, there are several causes of chronic cholestatic jaundice that one needs to consider. In addition to etiologies independent of HIV, including alcohol, primary sclerosing cholangitis (PSC), primary biliary cirrhosis (PBC), and sarcoidosis, there are several unique causes in those with HIV that must be considered (Table 17-1). Although HIV medications can be associated with

Table 17-1

Cause of Jaundice in the HIV Positive Patient

Common Causes	*Unique to HIV*
	Cholestatic Pattern
Gallstones	HIV medications
Sarcoidosis	Mycobaterium avium intracellulare
Primary biliary cirrhosis	Mycobacterium tuberculosis
Primary sclerosing cholangitis	HIV cholangiopathy
Alcohol	Papillary stenosis
Steatohepatitis	Bacillary angiomatosis
Cirrhosis	Lymphoma
Hepatocellular carcinoma	Kaposi's sarcoma
	Hepatocellular Pattern
Hepatitis A (acute)	HIV medications
Hepatitis B (acute or chronic, with or without	CMV
hepatitis D)	Herpes virus
Hepatitis C (chronic)	
Alcohol	
Steatohepatitis	
Vascular thrombosis	
Ischemia/hypoperfusion	
Cirrhosis	
Alpha-1 antitrypsin deficiency	
Wilson's disease	
Hemochromatosis	
	Normal Liver Enzymes
Gilbert's	Medication induced
	Indinavir
	Atazanavir

both acute and chronic increased alkaline phosphatase, jaundice is uncommon in the current era and highly active antiretroviral therapy (HAART) hepatotoxicity causing jaundice should be a diagnosis of exclusion. In those with poorly controlled HIV (low CD4 count and high HIV RNA level), opportunistic infections such as *Mycobacterium avium intracellulare* (MAI) and *Mycobacterium tuberculosis* (mTB) should be considered. Other unique causes of cholestasis in those with poorly controlled HIV include bacillary angiomatosis, lymphoma, Kaposi's sarcoma and HIV cholangiopathy, a disease that resembles PSC. With improved HIV therapy, HIV cholangiopathy is now rarely seen but has been linked to cytomegalovirus (CMV) and cryptosporidia. Papillary stenosis can also cause severe cholestasis in those with poorly controlled HIV, although jaundice is rarely seen. In evaluating cholestasis in the HIV patient, magnetic resonance imaging with cholangiography (MRI/MRCP) will often help guide the evaluation and liver biopsy can often be avoided.

The approach to the HIV patient with hepatocellular injury (increased aminotransferases) associated with jaundice should be similar to those without HIV; however, there are unique characteristics in the HIV patient to consider. Due to shared routes of transmission, coinfection with hepatitis C virus (HCV) and hepatitis B virus (HBV) is common and increases the risk of HAART hepatotoxicity. Furthermore, hepatic fibrosis may be accelerated in those with coinfection and once cirrhosis develops, decompensation may progress at a faster rate. Also, development of hepatocellular carcinoma (HCC) in those with cirrhosis may be higher in patients with HIV and should be considered in any patient with cirrhosis who develops jaundice. In selected candidates, liver transplantation should be considered and patients referred to appropriate centers.

Due to higher risk life styles, alcohol and acute viral hepatitis A or B should be strongly considered as the cause of jaundice in any HIV patient. In addition, since chronic HBV is seen in 5% to 10% of those living with HIV, seroconversion from HBe antigen to HBe antibody, seroreversion, or superinfection with hepatitis D should also be considered. Acute hepatitis C causing jaundice is rare but has been seen. Perhaps one of the most common causes of jaundice in those with HIV is benign elevations in unconjugated bilirubin due to inhibition of UDP-glucuronyl transferase. Both indinavir and atazanavir have both been associated with a similar clinical picture to Gilbert's syndrome. Although total bilirubin elevations are usually mild, they can approach 6 mg/dL. Because this can also occur in those with established cirrhosis, it is important to fractionate the bilirubin to differentiate this benign condition from true hepatic decompensation.

Once these more common causes of jaundice are excluded, other less common causes of chronic liver disease unique to HIV should be ruled out (Table 17-1). HIV medications have been associated with marked increased transaminases (grade 3 and 4: >5-10× upper limit of normal) and have led to the development of jaundice. Antiretroviral medications can cause severe hepatic dysfunction from a variety of mechanisms including direct hepatotoxicity and mitochondrial dysfunction associated with severe steatosis (see Table 14-1). NRTIs and protease inhibitors (PIs) have both been linked to the development of insulin resistance and dyslipidemia, conditions commonly associated with hepatic steatosis. Although high-dose ritonavir has been associated with grade 3 and 4 hepatotoxicity, current antiretroviral regimens that include a PI with "boosted ritonavir" are less of a contributing factor. Most studies have shown that those coinfected with HBV or HCV are at higher risk for severe hepatotoxicity from antiretroviral medications. If jaundice with elevations in liver enzymes is present, consultation from an infectious disease specialist and consideration of discontinuing antiretroviral medications is recommended.

In summary, the approach to the HIV patient with jaundice should first focus on determining whether it is related to liver disease. Those with isolated elevations in unconjugated bilirubin and normal liver enzymes on indinavir or atazanavir can be followed conservatively and often require no action. If severe liver dysfunction is present (coagulopathy and encephalopathy) in the absence of known liver disease, acute liver failure should be suspected and may require hospitalization. In those with intact synthetic function, I would next look at the pattern of liver injury. In those with acute cholestasis, I recommend liver imaging with ultrasound for evaluation of bile duct dilatation or mass. If evidence of biliary obstruction is seen, ERCP may be required. If there are no dilated ducts, then consider MRI/MRCP and proceed with excluding common conditions and those unique to HIV (Table 17-1). In those with chronic liver disease, the most common causes of jaundice are alcohol and viral hepatitis; however, other less common causes of chronic liver disease should also be excluded. Severe hepatotoxicity from antiretroviral medications can occur but is a diagnosis of exclusion. In cases of doubt, liver biopsy can sometimes be helpful in excluding chronic conditions and assessing the cause of injury. HIV patients with acute or chronic liver disease and severe hepatic dysfunction should be referred to liver centers that offer transplantation to those with HIV. With a rational approach, the HIV patient who develops jaundice can be managed with confidence.

References

1. Schneiderman DJ, Arenson DM, Cello JP, Margaretten W, Weber TE. Hepatic disease in patients with the acquired immune deficiency syndrome (AIDS). *Hepatology.* 1987;7:925-930.
2. Sulkowski MS, Thomas MS, Chaisson RE, Moore RD. Hepatotoxicity associated with antiretroviral therapy in adults infected with human immunodeficiency virus and the role of hepatitis C or B virus infection. *JAMA.* 2000;283:74-80.
3. Spengler U, Lichterfeld M, Rockstroh JK. Antiretroviral drug toxicity—a challenge for the hepatologist? *J Hepatol.* 2002;36:283-294.
4. Thomas DL. Growing importance of liver disease in HIV-infected persons. *Hepatology.* 2006;43:S221-S229.
5. Puoti M, Torti C, Ripamonti D, et al. Severe hepatoxicity during combination antiretroviral treatment: incidence, liver histology, and outcome. *J Acquir Immune Defic Syndr.* 2003;32:259-267.
6. Dieterich DT, Robinson PA, Lover J, Stern JO. Drug-induced liver injury associated with the use of nonnucleoside reverse-transcriptase inhibitors. *Clin Infect Dis.* 2004;38(suppl 2):S80-S89.
7. Sulkowski MS. Drug-induced liver injury associated with antiretroviral therapy that includes HIV-1 protease inhibitors. *Clin Infect Dis.* 2004;38(suppl 2):S90-S97.
8. Sulkowski MS, Mehta SH, Chaisson RE, Thomas DL, Moore RD. Hepatotoxicity associated with protease inhibitor-based antiretroviral regimens with or without concurrent ritonivir. *AIDS.* 2004;18:2277-2284.
9. Wit FWNM, Weverling GJ, Weel J, Jurriaans S, Lange JMA. Incidence of and risk factors for severe hepatotoxicity associated with antiretroviral combination therapy. *J Infect Dis.* 2002;186:23-31.
10. Bruno R, Sacchi P, Maiocchi L, Zocchetti C, Filice G. Hepatotoxicity and nelfinavir: A meta-analysis. *Clin Gastroenterol Hepatol.* 2005;3:482-488.
11. Mehta SH, Thomas DL, Torbenson M, Brinkley S, Mirel L, et al. The effect of antiretroviral therapy on liver disease among adults with HIV and hepatitis C coinfection. *Hepatology.* 2005;41;123-131.

SHOULD I STOP HIV MEDICATIONS IN A PATIENT WHO HAS DEVELOPED AN ELEVATION IN SERUM TRANSAMINASES?

Richard K. Sterling, MD, MSc, FACP, FACG

With the advent of highly active antiretroviral therapy (HAART), which combines various nucleoside/nucleotide analogue reverse transcriptase inhibitors (NRTIs), non-nucleoside reverse transcriptase inhibitors (NNRTIs), and protease inhibitors (PIs), the morbidity and mortality related to human immunodeficiency virus (HIV) have significantly decreased. As a result, patients are now living longer with HIV infection and other comorbidities and hepatic events have emerged as a key issue in the management of HIV-infected patients.[1,2]

Before you consider what to do in the HIV patient with elevated liver enzymes, you must first understand the problem. Abnormal liver chemistries (aspartate aminotransferase, AST; alanine aminotransferase, ALT; and alkaline phosphatase, ALP) are common and occur in 40% to 60% of patients on current HAART regimens even in the absence of hepatitis C virus (HCV) or hepatitis B virus (HBV), and their management remains a challenge. This high proportion of elevated liver enzymes is far greater than the 8% that occurs in the general population. According to the NIH-NAIA Guidelines from the AIDS Clinical Trial Group as shown in Table 18-1, elevations in liver enzymes are used to assess the grade of hepatoxicity. Of note, the grade is independently defined in those who have elevations of liver enzymes at baseline.

Increased liver enzymes in those with HIV may be due to a variety of factors, including viral hepatitis coinfections, HIV itself, alcohol, opportunistic infections, steatohepatitis, and concomitant medications including HAART (Figure 18-1). There have been several reports on hepatotoxicity related to HAART.[3-9] Most studies have focused on severe enzyme elevations (grades 3 to 4) and found an overall prevalence of 5% to 30% and higher in those coinfected with HCV or HBV. However, the majority of patients with abnormal liver chemistries have mild to moderate liver enzyme

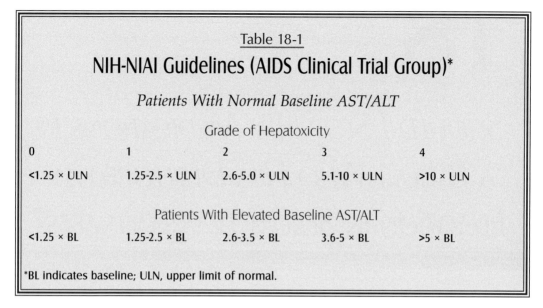

Table 18-1

NIH-NIAI Guidelines (AIDS Clinical Trial Group)*

Patients With Normal Baseline AST/ALT

Grade of Hepatoxicity

0	1	2	3	4
<1.25 × ULN	1.25-2.5 × ULN	2.6-5.0 × ULN	5.1-10 × ULN	>10 × ULN

Patients With Elevated Baseline AST/ALT

<1.25 × BL	1.25-2.5 × BL	2.6-3.5 × BL	3.6-5 × BL	>5 × BL

*BL indicates baseline; ULN, upper limit of normal.

Figure 18-1. Causes for increased liver enzymes in those with HIV.

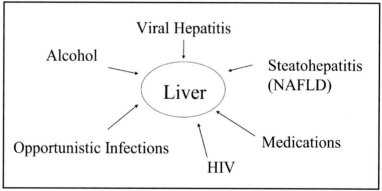

elevations (1.25-4× upper limit of normal, ULN). Because this group of patients has largely been ignored, especially in the absence of HCV or HBV, there are little data in these individuals without viral hepatitis who develop mild to moderate elevations in liver enzymes. In a recent report in a large cohort of 5957 HIV patients, the prevalence of abnormal ALT and AST (defined as greater than upper limit of normal) in those without HCV (n = 3997) was lower (55% and 76%, respectively) than those with HCV coinfection (83% for ALT and 92% for AST).[10] Importantly, 86% of these patients without HCV were also HBV surface antigen negative, suggesting another etiology for increased liver enzymes. Of those without HCV, 53% were on HAART and another 30% were on antiretrovirals of some sort. However, analyses for other factors associated with increased liver enzymes were not performed. Conversely, in a study by Maida and colleagues,[11] cryptogenic liver disease, defined as increased liver enzymes in the absence of HCV and HBV coinfections, was identified in only 17 of 3200 (0.5%) HIV-positive subjects. However, they excluded patients with severe obesity, grade 3 to 4 dyslipidemias, hyperglycemia, insulin resistance, and/or ultrasonographic evidence of fatty liver. Interestingly, even in the absence of risk for hepatic steatosis, liver histology in 5 demonstrated steatosis and inflammation. In their analysis, only longer didanosine (ddI) exposure was identified as an independent predictor of chronic liver enzyme elevations.

We recently looked at over 1200 unselected HIV patients to quantify the prevalence and factors associated with elevated LFTs.[12] The mean age was 42 years, 63% were male, 25% were Caucasian, and 22% had a BMI > 30. Overall, 24% had antibodies to HCV, 7.1% were positive for HBV surface antigen, and 1% was positive for both HCV and HBV. Of the cohort, 66% were taking HAART. Of these on HAART, 99%, 41.3%, and 59% were on a NRTI, NNRTI, and PI, respectively. Elevated AST, ALT, and ALP were observed in 31.5%, 23.8%, and 46.9% of the entire cohort. The overwhelming majority of elevations in liver enzymes were mild to moderate grade 1 to 2, with only 1% to 2% having elevations greater than 5× ULN (grades 3 to 4). Because HCV and HBV coinfection was the strongest predictor of abnormal liver enzymes in the entire cohort, possibly masking other factors, we focused on the risk factors of abnormal liver enzymes in those without HCV and HBV. In this group (n = 679), increased AST, ALT, and ALP were observed in 134 (19.7%), 103 (15.1%), and 291 (42.8%), respectively.

The causes of increased liver enzymes can include direct cytopathic effects of HIV on either hepatocytes or biliary epithelia or specific drug toxicity of HAART. There are several potential mechanisms that are specific to HIV medications that can result in liver enzyme elevations.[13] Restoration of the immune system with initiation of antiretroviral therapy has been associated with worsening of underlying infections, such as HCV and HBV. PIs have been associated with the development of insulin resistance (IR) and dyslipidemia, both risk factors for steatosis, which often present as asymptomatic liver enzyme elevations and may explain elevations in liver enzymes in some of these individuals. The prevalence of steatosis in those with HIV is unknown in those without HCV coinfection. Several recent reports in HIV-HCV coinfected patients have found a high proportion (40 to 75%) with steatosis that is greater than expected from the general population and associated with increased weight, hyperglycemia, lipodystrophy, stavudine, NRTI, and PI use. Therefore, the ability of HAART and other drugs to disrupt the normal production or elimination of reactive oxygen species in the liver may be an important factor relating to their potential cause of abnormal liver enzymes.

Because the majority of liver enzyme increases are mild, no specific action is required. If the elevations are new and persistent, other causes of chronic liver disease should be excluded including alcohol and viral hepatitis. In those few that develop severe elevations (grades 3 and 4) and jaundice, consideration of discontinuing HAART should be made after consultation with an infectious disease specialist. The decision to restart antiretroviral therapy and which medications to include can be difficult and depends on the need to suppress HIV and existing viral resistance. In those who fail to normalize enzymes after discontinuation, liver biopsy can be considered to establish the severity of underlying liver disease. Those with active HCV or HBV should be referred for antiviral therapy (see Questions on HIV-HCV and HIV-HBV for more details). If steatosis is present, I would assess for IR and dyslipidemia and consider changing to another regimen that will be effective in controlling HIV.

Bibliography

1. Schneiderman DJ, Arenson DM, Cello JP, Margaretten W, Weber TE. Hepatic disease in patients with the Acquired Immune Deficiency Syndrome (AIDS). *Hepatology*. 1987;7:925-930.
2. Thomas DL. Growing importance of liver disease in HIV-infected persons. *Hepatology*. 2006;43:S221-S229.
3. Sulkowski MS, Mehta SH, Chaisson RE, Thomas DL, Moore RD. Hepatotoxicity associated with protease inhibitor-based antiretroviral regimens with or without concurrent ritonavir. *AIDS*. 2004;18(17):2277-2284.
4. Sulkowki MS, Thomas MS, Chaisson RE, Moore RD. Hepatotoxicity associated with antiretroviral therapy in adults infected with human immunodeficiency virus and the role of hepatitis C or B virus infection. *JAMA*. 2000;283:74-80.
5. Puoti M, Torti C, Ripamonti D, et al. Severe hepatotoxicity during combination antiretroviral treatment: incidence, liver histology, and outcome. *J Acquir Immune Defic Syndr*. 2003; 32(3):259-267.
6. Wit FWNM, Weverling GJ, Weel J, Jurriaans S, Lange JMA. Incidence of and risk factors for severe hepatotoxicity associated with antiretroviral combination therapy. *JID*. 2002;186:23-31.
7. Bruno R, Sacchi P, Maiocchi L, Zocchetti C, Filice G. Hepatotoxicity and nelfinavir: A meta-analysis. *Clin Gastroenterol Hepatol*. 2005;3:482-488.
8. Spengler U, Lichterfeld M, Rockstroh JK. Antiretroviral drug toxicity – a challenge for the hepatologist? *J Hepatology* 2002;36:283-294.
9. Neff GW, Jayawerra D, Sherman KE. Drug-induced liver injury in HIV Patients. *Gastroenterol Hepatol*. 2006; 2:430-437
10. Rockstroh JK, Mocroft A, Soriano V, et al. Influence of hepatitis C virus infection on HIV-1 disease progression and response to highly active antiviral therapy. *J Infect Dis*. 2005;192:992-1002.
11. Maida I, Nunez M, Rios MJ, et al. Severe liver disease associated with prolonged exposure to antiretroviral drugs. *JAIDS*. 2006;42:177-182.
12. Sterling RK, Chui S, Snider K, Nixon D. The prevalence and risk factors for abnormal liver enzymes in HIV-positive patients without hepatitis B or C coinfections. *Digest Dis Sci*. 2008 (in press).
13. Pol S, Lebray P, Vallet-Pichard A. HIV infection and hepatic enzyme abnormalities: intricacies of the pathogenic mechanisms. *Clin Infect Dis*. 2004;38 Suppl 2:S65-S72.

SECTION IV

GENETIC DISORDERS THAT CAUSE CHRONIC LIVER DISEASE

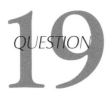
WHAT IS THE BEST SCREENING TEST FOR GENETIC HEMOCHROMATOSIS?

Peter Dienhart, MD
Jayanta Choudhury, MD
Anastasios A. Mihas, MD, DMSc, FACP, FACG

Introduction

Hereditary hemochromatosis (HH) is an inherited disorder of iron metabolism that leads to excess parenchymal iron deposition in various organs of the body. Although originally described in the early 1800s, the genetic basis was deciphered only in the mid-1990s and linked to the HFE (hemochromatosis) gene attached to the short arm of chromosome 6. It also happens to be one of the most common inherited disorders that lead to chronic liver disease in patients of northern European descent. HH, if diagnosed early, is a preventable etiology of chronic liver disease. As cirrhosis continues to be the 10th leading cause of death in United States, it is critically important to ensure effective screening and early diagnosis of HH.[1]

Disorders of Iron Overload

Although the pathophysiologic end point of all iron overload states involves excess iron in the tissue parenchyma eventually leading to organ dysfunction, it is important to distinguish the primary from the secondary iron overload states. Primary iron overload states, including all genetic disorders of iron metabolism, lead to increased iron absorption and subsequent deposition in various organs including the liver, pancreas, pituitary, heart, testes, skin, and bones. The most common of this group of disorders is the HFE gene–related HH, while others include disorders affecting the iron transporters (transferrin, ferroportin), the African iron overload states, and juvenile hemochromatosis.

HFE gene–related HH has been linked with two genetic mutations, C282Y and H63D. The presence of these mutations in both alleles of the HFE gene confers an increased risk of developing parenchymal iron overload. However, the phenotypic expression of this disorder is not always guaranteed by the presence of these mutations, even in the homozygous state. Thus, to be clinically significant, the genetic abnormalities have to come together with both increased body iron levels and actual involvement of target organs. However, the long-term prognosis in individuals with HFE gene mutations, normal iron studies, and no apparent target organ damage is unclear.

Due to the remarkable heterogeneity of presentation of HH and overall clinical outcomes, it is important to separate it from conditions that lead to excess iron stores and eventual deposition in target organs. The most common of these secondary iron overload states are the chronic hemolytic anemias, porphyria cutanea tarda (PCT), and various other chronic liver diseases such as alcoholic liver disease, chronic hepatitis C, and fatty liver disease. The pattern of hepatic iron in primary and secondary iron overload disorders differ, with the former having predominantly iron deposition in the hepatocytes and the latter targeting the hepatic sinusoidal or Kuppfer cells. This pattern recognition may be important in patients in whom diagnosis is confounded by the presence of more than one etiologic association.

Role of Iron Studies in Screening for Iron Overload States

To be effective, a screening strategy has to have the ability to distinguish primary from secondary iron overload states and to identify those individuals at higher risk for iron-induced organ damage. The workup at presentation, of all patients with suspected chronic liver disease that fit the demographic profile, should include an iron panel and serum ferritin levels.[2] While it is well recognized that iron levels in patients with HFE mutations may be normal, it is also less likely that a patient who has cirrhosis due to untreated HH will have normal iron levels. It is also noteworthy that although serum ferritin is an acute-phase reactant and is frequently elevated in patients with acute disease states, it is less common to find levels >1000 µg/L, along with other iron markers, in patients without HH. The other indicators of excess iron levels that are used to screen patients with suspected HH include transferrin saturation, serum iron, and iron binding capacity. In a large national study (HEIRS study), looking at screening for HH, it was found that patients with HFE gene mutations had higher levels of iron markers compared to their counterparts without the HFE mutation.[3] It was also found that patients with homozygous C282Y mutations had the highest ferritin levels and transferrin saturations, followed by compound heterozygotes (C282Y/H63D combination). These individuals usually had high ferritin levels >1000 µg/L and transferrin saturation >50%. There is also a variation in the serum ferritin levels among males and females who have mutations for the HFE gene, with females generally having lower levels compared to matched male cohorts.

In patients with secondary iron overload states, such as chronic hemolytic anemias and other chronic liver diseases, it is not uncommon to find abnormal iron studies and target organ deposition of iron. Studies looking at the possible role of iron in the pathogenesis of chronic hepatitis C have found that between 30% and 60% of patients with chronic hepatitis C may have abnormal serum ferritin and/or serum transferrin saturation. Similarly, abnormal iron studies and isolated copies of HFE gene mutations have been found in a subset of patients with fatty liver disease and some studies have suggested that these groups of patients may have increased fibrosis, but this conclusion has not been validated by other studies. The situation in alcoholic liver disease is different, with a significant proportion of patients having a modest degree of iron overload without any correlation with the HFE gene mutation. Moreover, these patients with iron overload do not show any increased progression to fibrosis or cirrhosis and most authorities now believe that presence of HFE gene mutation in this subset of patients has no pathogenic effect.

In summary, iron studies are sensitive biochemical markers to screen for patients with iron overload states. Routine preliminary workup of patients presenting to a gastroenterologist for the first time with suspected liver disease should include iron studies, serum ferritin levels and transferrin saturation. The drawback of iron studies is the lack of specificity although the presence of very high serum ferritin (>1000 µg/L) and transferrin (>50%) levels in an appropriate clinical setting makes it a useful diagnostic tool. Once the clinical suspicion of iron overload state is aroused, one should proceed accordingly to the more definitive tests before making the final diagnosis of HH.

ROLE OF GENETIC TESTING IN THE SCREENING OF IRON OVERLOAD STATES

The definitive diagnosis of HH is based on the detection of HFE gene mutations. Hence, the older diagnostic algorithm based on liver biopsy findings of stainable iron in the hepatocytes with clinical and biochemical correlation of iron overload is no longer valid in most situations. The two common mutations that are detected include C282Y and H63D. The prevalence of HFE gene mutations was assessed in a large study of 99 711 individuals diagnosed with iron overload state; 299 of them were homozygotes for the C282Y mutation.[4] Of these homozygous patients, 281 were non-Hispanic Whites (0.44% of total study group) followed by Hispanics and Asians. The disease phenotype in patients with homozygous H63D mutations is milder compared to C282Y mutations. In a smaller subgroup of patients, both the C282Y and H63D mutations may be present at the same time, lending the term *compound homozygotes*. These patients have a more severe iron overload state with more likely phenotypic display of overt disease. There have been other mutations such as S65C that have been detected either alone or in combination with other HFE gene mutations. While some of these mutations may produce overt disease, routine testing is usually not available outside research settings and is probably unnecessary to consider it as a part of the workup.

In summary, the definitive diagnosis of HH is dependent on the presence of HFE gene mutations in an appropriate clinical setting. The two common mutations available for testing are the C282Y and H63D; testing should be carried out in patients who have elevated iron levels on initial screening. Almost 85% of patients around the world and in the United States with HH have C282Y mutations and tend to have overt disease process involving the liver or other organs. The significance of one allelic mutation (heterozygous state) in the absence of other risk factors of chronic liver disease is probably clinically insignificant. However, concomitant hepatic injury either due to hepatitis and/or exposure to other potential hepatotoxins may put these heterozygous patients at increased risk for developing accelerated hepatic damage.

Table 19-1

Screening Tools for Hemochromatosis

Screening Test	*Comment*
Transferrin saturation (>50%)	Fasting serum levels have the greatest predictive value
Serum ferritin (>300 µg/L)	Low specificity, acute phase reactant Most common worldwide
HFE gene C282Y mutation H63D mutation	More potent phenotypic expression in compound heterozygous state (C282Y/H63D)
Liver biopsy: Hepatic Iron Index (HII, >1.9)	Invasive, expensive, sampling error Low sensitivity, low specificity
Computed tomography Magnetic resonance	Safer and less costly than LBx
SQUID*	High sensitivity; still experimental

*SQUID indicates Superconducting Quantum Interference Device.

ROLE OF LIVER BIOPSY IN IRON OVERLOAD STATES

Although liver biopsy is the most accurate method for assessing hepatic iron burden, its role in the initial diagnostic evaluation of HH has changed over the past few decades.[5] Characteristically, in HH the iron accumulates within the hepatocytes rather than in hepatic sinusoidal lining and Kuppfer cells as in secondary iron overload states. Hepatic iron concentration and the hepatic iron index (HII; hepatic iron concentration corrected for the patient's age) in liver biopsy specimens are useful indicators if the diagnosis of HFE cannot be made by genetic testing. Typically, cirrhosis is uncommon with hepatic iron concentrations below 16 000 µg/g dry weight in the absence of concomitant liver disease of other etiologies. It is at present extremely uncommon to use liver biopsy as an initial aid to diagnose or stratify HH, unless it is being done to assess the stage of hepatic damage.

In summary, it is currently unnecessary to obtain a liver biopsy for the diagnosis of HH unless it is being used as an assessment tool to detect the extent of hepatic damage. In fact, the current trend is to enhance the role of several noninvasive screening tools, some of which appear to be very promising (Table 19-1). It is obvious that if liver biopsy is done, then hepatic iron concentration should be measured for the accurate assessment of the extent of iron loading.

SCREENING OF THE FAMILY IN HH

HH is an autosomal recessive disease that is transmitted in a familial manner. Hence, genetic testing should be offered to first-degree relatives of patients with homozygous C282Y or H63D mutations and to those with compound C282Y/H63D heterozygous state. If the first-degree relative of the proband has either of these mutations and/or elevated iron levels, then prophylactic therapy should be considered. For children of patients with HH, both parents should have genetic analysis. If one parent has no mutations on the HFE gene, then the child is going to be heterozygote by definition and no further testing is required for the child. In contrast, if both parents have the mutations in either homozygous or heterozygous state, genetic testing should be done to characterize the risk of an iron overload state.

In conclusion, all patients who are assessed for abnormal liver function tests should be screened for iron overload states as early detection of HH can potentially prevent its effect on target organs. Once the diagnosis is suspected, based on iron studies, patients should undergo genetic testing to confirm the diagnosis. Liver biopsy is not necessary unless it is used for staging, for the assessment of the extent of hepatic damage, or for the elimination of other etiologies. Once the proband is identified, all first-degree relatives should be screened and if an HFE mutation is identified, early initiation of therapy will surely prevent target organ damage.

References

1. Dubois S, Kowdley KV. The importance of screening for hemochromatosis. *Arch Intern Med.* 2003;163: 2424-2426.
2. Qaseem A, Aronson M, Fitterman N, et al. Screening for hereditary hemochromatosis: a clinical practice guideline from the American College of Physicians. *Ann Intern Med.* 2005;143:517-521
3. Bacon BR. Screening for hemochromatosis. *Arch Intern Med.* 2006;166:269-270.
4. Whitlock EP, Garlitz BA, Harris EL. Screening for hereditary hemochromatosis: A systematic review for the US preventive services task force. *Ann Intern Med.* 2006;145:209-223.
5. Adams PC, Passmore L, Chakrabarti S, et al. Liver disease in the hemochromatosis and iron overload screening study. *Clin Gastroenterol Hepatol.* 2006;4:918-923.

How Frequently Should I Have a Patient With Genetic Hemochromatosis Undergo Phlebotomy?

Peter Dienhart, MD
Jayanta Choudhury, MD
Anastasios A. Mihas, MD, DMSc, FACP, FACG

Introduction

Hereditary hemochromatosis (HH) is one of the most common inherited causes of chronic liver disease, whose effects on target organs are preventable if detected early. Thus, the goal of treatment is the prevention of iron deposition in target organs as well as early treatment of its complications. Once the diagnosis is established, the therapeutic options are simple, effective, and relatively inexpensive.

Phlebotomy and HH

The most effective available therapeutic option to manage iron overload is phlebotomy.[1] It should be initiated in patients who are homozygous to the C282Y mutation, compound heterozygotes, and in any heterozygous individual with significant biochemical/histological evidence of iron overload. From the standpoint of liver disease, the ultimate aim is the prevention of cirrhosis and its complications in the genetically susceptible host. This becomes critically important because the leading cause of death in this cohort is hepatocellular carcinoma and, more often than not, complications of chronic liver disease bring these patients to the forefront of clinical care.

Phlebotomy should be initiated as soon as the diagnosis is made and 1 to 2 units of blood (1 unit of blood/500 mL = ~250 mg of iron) should be removed every week.[2] The aim of phlebotomy is to prevent the development of iron deficiency anemia while at the

<table>
<tr><td colspan="2" align="center">Table 20-1</td></tr>
<tr><td colspan="2" align="center">**Treatment of Hemochromatosis**</td></tr>
</table>

Therapeutic Modality	*Comment*
A. Hereditary hemochromatosis	
Phlebotomy	
Quantity of removed blood	˜500 mL
Frequency	Weekly to biweekly
Monitors	Ht prior to each phlebotomy (no phlebotomy if Ht drops >20%)
Goal	Serum ferritin <50 ng/mL
Avoid vitamin C supplements	Accelerates iron absorption and mobilization
Liver transplantation	Associated with high morbidity and mortality
B. Secondary iron overload	
Iron chelating agents	Desferioxamine (Desferal) 20 to 40 mg/kg
Avoid vitamin C	As above
Liver biopsy	To assess adequacy of iron removal

same time depleting the iron stores to normal or low normal levels. Usually, the patient with HH will have total body iron stores in excess of 30 g, and to deplete this to an acceptable level without initiating iron deficiency anemia takes anywhere from 2 to 3 years or more. During this period, iron indices including serum ferritin and transferrin saturation should be monitored as surrogate markers of body iron stores. However, it is probably unnecessary to initiate the measurement of either of these markers on a routine basis until about 5 to 6 weeks of regular phlelobotomy from the time of initiation. Serum transferrin saturation usually does not change until all body stores of iron are depleted. In contrast, serum ferritin levels are more variable, with decrease occurring once the iron stores have decreased below a certain critical level. Phlebotomy should be continued on a regular basis until the serum ferritin falls below 50 ng/mL and at that point maintenance phlebotomy initiated to maintain the serum ferritin levels between 25 and 50 ng/mL. The frequency and the need for maintenance phlebotomy are variable and may range from monthly to several times per year or even less. Serum ferritin levels should be allowed to fall below 25 ng/mL as iron deficiency anemia develops and complicates the management. The other index that is closely followed with every phlebotomy is hematocrit, and the phlebotomy process should not lead to drop in hematocrit values greater than 20% of baseline (Table 20-1).

The role of phlebotomy in preventing iron-induced damage to the liver, heart, pancreas, and the skin is well recognized. The initiation of phlebotomy may also decrease the systemic complaints of pain, fatigue, malaise, and, in some cases, skin pigmentation. It also has a role in decreasing the insulin requirements in established HH-related diabetics. However, its effectiveness in the prevention or amelioration of joint symptoms and hypogonadism is limited.

Management of HH-Related Chronic Liver Disease

In patients with established cirrhosis or bridging fibrosis, the role of phlebotomy in slowing the progression and/or reversal of changes is less certain. There is, however, a general consensus that phlebotomy should be initiated whenever the changes of chronicity are less prominent and the patient is otherwise able to tolerate phlebotomy. It is also important to note that although hepatocellular carcinoma (HCC) is rare in patients with HH without evidence of cirrhosis, several case reports have been reported in the literature. Hence, every effort should be made to exclude the presence of iron-induced liver damage, failing which HCC screening should be initiated. The cost-benefit ratio of screening for HCC in non-cirrhotic patients is unclear and it is also unknown whether the rare patients that develop HCC in the absence of cirrhosis have a different disease course. Hence, current guidelines do not recommend screening of patients with HH for HCC in the absence of cirrhosis.

In the unfortunate event that a patient does develop cirrhosis secondary to HH, orthotopic liver transplantation may be considered.[3] However, it should be borne in mind that these patients have a worse outcome compared to patients transplanted for cirrhosis of other etiologies. This is true even for patients who have been transplanted after adequate depletion of body iron stores. The most common reasons for this adverse outcome are postoperative cardiac dysfunction and infection-related complications that occur at a higher frequency in this cohort of patients. One of the explanations that have been offered for this paradigm is that despite overt depletion of body iron stores, the deposited parenchymal iron persists, especially in the heart, leading to postoperative cardiac decompensation and/or sudden death.

Adjunctive Therapies in HH

Since iron absorption from the gut is accelerated in HH, it is apparent that all medications known to increase iron absorption or mobilization should be avoided. One of the common medications that has been implicated in accelerated iron mobilization is vitamin C. This phenomenon is particularly important during the initiation of phlebotomy when there is rapid mobilization of iron from the body stores into the circulation. The presence of vitamin C in the circulation during this period accelerates the mobilization to the extent that all available transferring receptors get saturated. As a direct consequence, excessive free iron becomes available with resultant pro-oxidant and free radical–induced tissue damage.

The role of iron chelating therapies in HH is limited. The two most common chelating medications have been desferrioxamine and deferiprone. While the former can be used only parenterally (usually subcutaneously), the latter can be given orally. These two agents have been used either singly or concurrently in the therapy of patients unable to tolerate phlebotomy. The two major disadvantages of the chelating agents are their high cost and side effects, with up to a third of patients discontinuing therapy due to adverse effects. Hence, iron chelation therapy should be limited only to patients with HH who have serious cardiovascular and/or hemodynamic issues preventing them from tolerating phlebotomy.

Management of Secondary Iron Overload States

Secondary iron overload states more commonly fall in the ambit of hematologists rather than the gastroenterologist. However, there are several chronic liver diseases such as chronic hepatitis C, alcoholic and nonalcoholic fatty liver disease, as well as porphyria cutanea tarda (PCT) with increased body iron stores. With the exception of porphyria cutanea tarda, the role of phlebotomy and/or iron chelation in all of these clinical entities is uncertain and it is not recommended. In PCT, phlebotomy is an extremely effective means in reducing the burden of disease on the liver and it is done following similar guidelines as those of HH. Phlebotomy is also effective in African iron overload state, a rare disorder seen in a specific geographic location.

By far, the most common group of patients suffering from secondary iron overload states are those with chronic hemolytic anemias who are consequently transfusion dependent.[4] Phlebotomy is not an option in the majority of these patients due to low or borderline low hematocrit. Iron chelation therapy is the mainstay of treatment in these patients. However, monitoring the extent of depletion of total body iron is problematic in these individuals and serum ferritin and/or transferrin saturation are unreliable indices of iron mobilization in this population. The only reliable index of total body iron is hepatic iron index, obtained from measuring the iron content in liver biopsy specimens.[5] Frequently, these patients require serial liver biopsies to document adequate body iron depletion. Patients with persistent iron overload may develop hepatic fibrosis and cirrhosis. Hence, the aim of iron chelation therapy should be to keep the hepatic iron content below 15 000 μg/gm of dry weight in order to prevent the development of liver damage. Vitamin C should also be avoided in these patients for similar reason to that of HH state.

In conclusion, the entire focus of management of HH is directed at the prevention of target organ damage. Phlebotomy is the single most effective therapy for HH and should be considered in all homozygotes and in those with biochemical evidence of iron overload. Early cirrhosis is not a contraindication for phlebotomy and in fact may help to slow the progression of liver damage. Because HCC and complications of cirrhosis account for approximately half the mortality and morbidity, they should be aggressively diagnosed and appropriately treated. Iron chelation therapy is reserved for patients unable to tolerate phlebotomy and in patients with secondary iron overload states.

References

1. Tavill A. AASLD guideline: diagnosis and management of hemochromatosis. *Hepatology.* 2001;33:1321.
2. Adams PC. Review article: the modern diagnosis and management of hemochromatosis. *Aliment Pharmacol Ther.* 2006;23:1681-1691.
3. Kowdley KV, Brandhagen DJ, Gish RG, et al. Survival after liver transplantation in patients with hepatic iron overload: the national hemochromatosis transplant registry. *Gastroenterology.* 2005;129:494-503.
4. Brittenham GM, Griffith PM, Nienhuis AW, et al. Efficacy of desferioxamine in preventing complications of iron overload in patients with thalassemia major. *N Engl J Med.* 1994;331:567-57.
5. Angelucci E, Brittenham GM, McLaren CE, et al. Hepatic iron concentration and total body iron stores in thalassemia major. *N Engl J Med.* 2000;343:327-333.

WHAT IS THE BEST SCREENING TEST FOR WILSON'S DISEASE?

Opang Cheung, MD
Anastasios A. Mihas, MD, DMSc, FACP, FACG

Wilson's disease (WD) is an autosomal recessive disorder of copper metabolism affecting approximately 1 in 30 000 in the Caucasian population. It is 4 times more common in women than in men. The specific mutations on disease gene ATP7B, a copper-transporting ATPase located on chromosome 13 at 13q14.3-q21.1, result in impaired incorporation of copper into ceruloplasmin and thereby decreased biliary excretion of copper. This eventually leads to a dramatic buildup of intracellular copper to toxic levels in the liver, brain, and other sites in the body. The diagnosis of WD, especially in the presymptomatic stage, can be challenging because its symptoms are often indistinguishable from other chronic liver diseases and may evolve slowly over time rather than appearing all at once.

The age of disease onset ranges from 3 to more than 50 years of age and the initial symptoms can be hepatic, neurological, psychiatric, or as an acute hemolytic crisis. Hepatic involvement almost never appears before the age of 4 years and usually occurs during the first 2 decades of life. WD can present in one of the following 4 clinical subtypes: acute hepatitis, acute-on-chronic hepatitis, chronic hepatitis, and fulminant Wilson's disease (FWD). Chronic and acute-on-chronic hepatitis are associated with persistent asymptomatic elevation of aminotransferase and progressive development of liver cirrhosis. Acute hepatitis occurs in 25% of patients with WD and, due to its brief and resolving nature, it rarely leads to investigation for WD. FWD is rare, with a fatal outcome unless emergency liver transplantation is performed. Neurologic and psychiatric signs and symptoms may predominate in older patients and range from behavioral changes and anxiety disorders to depression and psychosis. WD must be considered in patients below the age of 40 years with unexplained liver disease or cirrhosis and in patients with neurological and psychiatric symptoms and evidence of concurrent liver disease.

Table 21-1

Clinical and Laboratory Manifestations of Wilson's Disease

Clinical

Hepatic
Fulminant hepatic failure
Acute autoimmune hepatitis
Autoimmune-like chronic active hepatitis
Cirrhosis
Compensated
Decompensated
Fatty liver
Asymptomatic hepatomegaly

Neuropsychiatric
Movement disorders (tremor, dystonia)
Dysarthria
Hypersalivation
Ataxic gait
Convulsions
Depression
Neuroses
Psychoses
Personality changes

Miscellaneous
Kayser-Fleischer rings
Keratitis
Arthritis
Bone deformities
Renal abnormalities
Cardiomyopathy

Laboratory

Biochemical
Elevated serum aminotransferases
Decreased serum ceruloplasmin
Low serum alkaline phosphatase
Increased serum copper
Increased urine copper excretion
Decreased serum uric acid (?)

Hematologic
Hemolytic anemia (Coombs-negative)
Thrombocytopenia
Increased unconjugated bilirubin
Hypoprothrombinemia

Histologic
Steatosis
Autoimmune-like CAH
Cirrhosis
Rhodamine stain
Increased liver copper concentration

The prognosis of WD depends on the extent of liver or nervous system damage before treatment. For those with advanced liver disease unresponsive to medical treatment, liver transplantation remains the only cure. It is therefore very important that patients with WD be diagnosed early and prior to any symptom development; hence the need for effective screening.

Clinical and laboratory parameters (Table 21-1) are not sufficient to exclude the diagnosis of WD in patients with liver disease of unknown origin. It is anticipated that the use of genetic testing and direct detection of the mutations causing WD will eliminate the difficulties in distinguishing presymptomatic patients from heterozygotes, although the gene is large and more than 250 mutations have already been identified. Fortunately, molecular diagnostic studies (DNA testing) have made it possible to define patterns of haplotypes or polymorphisms of DNA surrounding the disease gene ATP78 and identify affected siblings of probands.

Table 21-2

Family Screening for Wilson's Disease*

- History
- Physical examination (including slit-lamp exam for K-F rings)
- Complete blood count (CBC)
- Serum aminotransferase levels
- Tests of hepatic synthetic function
- Serum ceruloplasmin levels
- Serum copper levels
- 24-H urinary copper excretion†
- Genetic tests
- Genotypes (cases with known mutations)
- Haplotypes

*Recommended for first-degree relatives (siblings) by the 2003 AASLD guideline.
†Proceed with liver biopsy if positive.

At present, no single test is able to identify affected siblings or heterozygote carriers of the WD gene with sufficient certainty. Based on the current American Association for the Study of Liver Disease (AASLD) guideline, it is recommended that all first-degree relatives of patients diagnosed with WD be screened by a combination of clinical findings and biochemical tests. Appropriate screening should include a history and physical examination, liver biochemical tests, complete blood count, serum ceruloplasmin (normal 20 to 40 mg/dL), slit-lamp examination for Kayser-Fleischer (KF) rings (often absent early on, present in 50% of patients with hepatic presentation but 98% of patients with neurological or psychiatric signs or symptoms), 24-h basal urinary copper determination (normal <50 µg/24 h > 100 µg/24 h in most symptomatic patients and following chelation therapy; <100 µg/24 h in patients on zinc therapy), and molecular studies with haplotype and mutation analysis as mentioned earlier. The first 4 tests (ie, history and physical, liver biochemical tests, complete blood count, and serum ceruloplasmin) are usually performed first and further testing is performed only in patients with suggestive features (Table 21-2).

In patients who are acutely ill or in newly diagnosed hepatic failure, the key is to quickly diagnose FWD from other etiologies of hepatic failure. FWD, although rapidly lethal without liver transplantation, can be managed successfully if early diagnosis is obtained. Patients with FWD typically have a nonimmune hemolytic anemia (due to the toxic hemolytic effects of copper), low alkaline phosphatase levels compared to total bilirubin (ratio < 4), aminotransferase <500 IU/L, hypoalbuminemia, and coagulopathy. In this setting, serum (>200 µg/dL), urine and hepatic copper concentration are markedly elevated. Hepatic copper normally is <40 µg/g dry weight liver; >250 µg/g dry weight liver is seen in most patients with WD. By contrast, serum ceruloplasmin, an acute-phase reactant, may even be elevated, thus leading to the erroneous exclusion of WD. Liver his-

> ### Table 21-3
> # Treatment of Wilson's Disease
>
> - D-penicillamine
> - Trientine (trien)
> - Ammonium tetrathiomolybdate (experimental)
> - Oral zinc
> - Antioxidants
> - Diet low in copper
> - Orthotopic liver transplantation

tology shows steatosis, glycogen nuclei, fibrosis, chronic hepatitis, and cirrhosis. Marked degeneration of hepatocytes, pleiocytosis, and nuclear irregularities are seen in cases of fulminant hepatitis.

Treatment of WD with zinc and the oral chelating agents penicillamine and trientine is lifelong. Liver transplantation and dietary restrictions are recommended along with medical therapy (Table 21-3). While awaiting a liver donor, the use of albumin dialysis, plasma exchange, or plasmapheresis will lower serum copper. Patients who survive beyond 1 year after liver transplantation have excellent long-term survival without disease recurrence.

References

1. Roberts EA, Schilsky ML. AASLD guideline: a practice guideline on Wilson's disease. *Hepatology.* 2003;37:1475-1487.
2. Gitlin JD. Wilson's disease. *Gastroenterology.* 2003;125:1868-1877.
3. Ala A, Schilsky ML. Wilson's disease; pathophysiology, diagnosis, treatment, and screening. *Clin Liver Dis.* 2004;8:787-805.
4. Ferenci P. Wilson's disease. *Clin Gastroenterol Hepatol.* 2005;3:726-733.
5. Brewer GJ, Askari FK. Wilson's disease: clinical management and therapy. *J Hepatol.* 2005;42:S13-S21.

WHAT SHOULD I TELL MY PATIENT WHO IS A CARRIER FOR ALPHA-1-ANTITRYPSIN DEFICIENCY?

Anastasios A. Mihas, MD, DMSc, FACP, FACG

Introduction

In 1963, Laurel and Eriksson first reported the presence of α1-antitrypsin (AAT) deficiency in young patients with pulmonary emphysema. In the late 1960s, Sharp and his coworkers described liver cirrhosis in 10 children with AAT deficiency. Today, we know that AAT deficiency is an autosomal recessive lethal hereditary disorder that affects 1 in 2500 individuals worldwide and is associated with a substantial risk for the development of pulmonary emphysema and liver cirrhosis. Unfortunately, AAT deficiency is clinically underdiagnosed, although it is the most common genetic liver disease in children and the leading cause for liver transplantation in this age group.

Pathogenesis of Liver Disease

AAT is a serum glycoprotein composed of 394 amino acids, which is coded by a single gene on the q arm of chromosome 14, which is a member of a family of serpins.[1] AAT is almost exclusively produced by the liver. Its main function, as an acute-phase reactant, is anti-protease activity against neutrophil proteases such as elastase, cathepsin G, and proteinase. The AT gene has an extensive polymorphism with more than 75 different alleles described thus far. The various alleles are assigned a letter code (A to Z) according to their electrophoretic mobility. The normal AAT alleles are referred to as M and are found in almost 90% of individuals of European origin. The most common deficient allele associated with liver disease is the Z allele, which is present in

Table 22-1			
Risk of Liver and Lung Disease **According to AAT Phenotype**			
Phenotype	*Risk for Liver Disease*	*Risk for Lung Disease*	*Serum AAT*
MM	No	No	Normal
MZ	Slightly increased	Slightly increased	Slightly decreased
SS	No	No	Normal
SZ	Slightly increased	Increased (20% to 30%)	Decreased
ZZ	High	High (85% to 100%)	<15%
Null	No	High (100% by 30th year)	0

less than 3% of Caucasians. This Z allele (ATZ) represents a mutant of the normal AAT gene allele (M), which triggers a series of events that are eventually hepatotoxic. More than 95% of individuals with severe AAT deficiency are homozygous for the Z allele (ie, PiZZ phenotype) and consequently at high risk for emphysema and liver disease (Table 22-1). The ATZ molecule's point mutation (substitution of lysine for glutamate) results in excessive transformation of the protein, which leads to increased concentration, temperature-dependent polymerization, and eventually intracellular degradation and accumulation within the hepatocyte. These intrahepatic inclusions have hepatotoxic effects, especially during septic or febrile episodes, which enhance polymerization and increase intracellular accumulation. This ATZ polymerization theory has been challenged recently by some investigators, who suggest that polymerization of ATZ is not the cause but rather the result of its retention by the endosplasmic reticulum (ER).

Clinical Manifestations

The main clinical manifestations of AAT deficiency pertain to three different organs: the lung (pulmonary emphysema), the liver (neonatal hepatitis, chronic active hepatitis, cirrhosis), and less frequently the skin (panniculitis).[2] In addition, there are some sporadic reports of several other conditions in association with AAT deficiency such as aneurysms, vasculitides, nephropathy, etc (Table 22-2).

Risk of Liver Disease in PiZZ Homozygotes

The association between AAT deficiency and liver disease was first observed in the late 1960s by Sharp and his colleagues. The typical patient is an elderly nonalcoholic male with negative hepatitis B and hepatitis C serology, presenting with cirrhosis or its complications, such as portal hypertension, or even hepatocellular carcinoma.

Table 22-2	
Clinical Manifestations of AAT Deficiency	
Manifestation	*Comment*
Lung disease	Early (premature) emphysema
	Panacinar emphysema
Liver disease	
Infants	Neonatal hepatitis
Children	Chronic active hepatitis
Adolescents, adults	Cryptogenic cirrhosis
	Portal hypertension
	Hepatocellular carcinoma
Dermatologic	
Necrotizing panniculitis	Third most common manifestation
Necrotizing vasculitides	Only 14 case reports
Systemic vasculitis	
Multiorgan vasculitides	Immune-mediated
Nephropathy	Various types of glomerulonephritis (children)
Miscellaneous	
Aneurysmal disease	Abdominal aorta, intracranial
Pancreatic disease	Exocrine and endocrine
Celiac disease	Weak evidence

In early childhood, approximately half of the PiZZ infants have abnormal liver enzymes but only a small number of them (<20%) develop clinical symptoms of liver disease.[3] By and large, more than 75% of the children will remain clinically healthy and with normal liver tests for most of their childhood and adolescence. Nonetheless, a significant number of the PiZZ children (~10%) will develop progressive liver disease with rapid decompensation, necessitating liver transplantation. If biliary atresia is excluded, AAT deficiency–induced end-stage liver disease (ESLD) accounts for 25% to 50% of all liver transplants in children and remains the most frequent genetic disorder that leads to chronic liver disease (CLD) and cirrhosis as well as the need for liver transplantation.

In the adult, the risk of PiZZ individuals for the development of chronic liver disease and cirrhosis increases significantly with aging.[4] Several case-control studies have established that while the risk of PiZZ homozygosity between 20 and 50 years of age is less than 2%, in patients over 50 years of age it is 10-fold higher (~20%). It is noteworthy that these individuals never smoked, thus surviving without developing pulmonary emphysema. With the exception of low serum AAT levels, all other clinical and laboratory findings of these patients are almost identical to those with cirrhosis of other etiologies. The risk of HCC is much higher than the risk for other chronic liver diseases and may even occur in the absence of cirrhosis.[5]

Risk of Liver Disease in PiZM Heterozygotes

The role of the heterozygous PiZ state (ie, phenotype PiZM) of AAT deficiency in the pathogenesis of chronic liver disease and cirrhosis is at best controversial.[6] To date, there has been no population study that assesses the risk of liver disease in adult patients with heterozygous AAT deficiency. Thus, it remains unclear whether heterozygous AAT deficiency is sufficient for the development of chronic liver disease and cirrhosis or whether additional factors are important.

In a recent US study, no association between PiZM of AAT and the presence of chronic liver or cirrhosis was found. In contrast, patients with decompensated cirrhosis of any etiology had a significantly higher prevalence of PiZM than their counterparts with fully compensated liver disease. The authors concluded that the PiZM AAT heterozygous state may have a role in the aggravation of liver disease due to either hepatitis C virus (HCV) or nonalcoholic fatty liver disease (NAFLD). Yet, the lack of large population-based prospective studies is an obvious limitation for a conclusive estimate of the propensity of AAT heterozygosity to develop chronic liver disease and cirrhosis. Several earlier studies suggested an increased risk for CLD and cirrhosis among AAT heterozygotes but most of them had several methodological flows such as small number of patients, high prevalence of cryptogenic cirrhosis, and, perhaps more importantly, were conducted prior to the recognition of HCV and NAFLD.

SO, WHAT SHOULD THE CLINICIAN TELL HIS PATIENT WHO IS HETEROZYGOUS FOR AAT DEFICIENCY?

Patients should know that at the present time there is no clear evidence that AAT heterozygosity predisposes to liver disease and cirrhosis or hepatocellular carcinoma. However, the presence of AAT heterozygosity in patients with CLD of other etiologies increases the risk for progressive liver disease and decompensation. For this reason, the World Health Organization recommends mandatory vaccination both for hepatitis A and hepatitis B of these individuals.

Treatment

To date, there is no specific treatment for AAT deficiency-associated liver disease. Perhaps the single most important supportive measure is cessation of smoking to prevent exacerbation of the lung disease. Several studies have shown that continued smoking accelerates the AAT deficiency–associated emphysema and leads to higher morbidity and mortality rates.

Contrary to the treatment of lung disease with the exogenous administration of recombinant AAT, such therapy is not recommended in patients with liver disease because its pathogenesis (excess of AAT) is exactly the opposite from that of lung disease (lack of AAT).

Liver transplantation remains the only definitive treatment of AAT deficiency–induced liver disease and is associated with over 90% 5-year survival. It should be kept in mind that a large number of children may have mild liver dysfunction and may never need transplantation. Furthermore, even those with advanced chronic liver disease and cirrhosis can lead a normal life for a long time without the need for liver transplantation. If liver transplantation is not possible, complications of cirrhosis should be managed as in any other chronic liver disease.

References

1. Perlmutter DH. The cellular basis for liver injury in α1-antitrypsin deficiency. *Hepatology.* 1991;172-185.
2. American Thoracic Society. ATS/ERS statement: standards for the diagnosis and management of individuals with AAT deficiency. I. Executive summary. *Am J Respir Crit Care Med.* 2003;168:818.
3. Perlmutter DH. Alpha-1-antitrypsin deficiency: diagnosis and treatment. *Clin Liver Dis.* 2004;8:839-859.
4. Bowlus CH, Willner I, Zern MA, et al. Factors associated with advanced liver disease in adults with alpha-1-antitrypsin deficiency. *Clin Gastroenterol Hepatol.* 2005;3:390-396.
5. Rudnick DA, Perlmutter DH. Alpha-1-antitrypsin deficiency: a new paradigm for hepatocellular carcinoma in genetic liver disease. *Hepatology.* 2005;42:514-521.
6. Regev A, Guaqueta C, Molina EG, et al. Does the heterozygous state of alpha-1-antitrypsin deficiency have a role in chronic liver diseases? Interim results of a large case-control study. *J Pediatr Gastroenterol Nutr.* 2006;1:S30-S35.

DO ALL PATIENTS WITH AUTOIMMUNE HEPATITIS REQUIRE IMMUNE SUPPRESSIVE MEDICATIONS?

R. Todd Stravitz, MD

Autoimmune hepatitis (AIH) has three clinical presentations: abnormal liver chemistries in an asymptomatic patient, acute icteric hepatitis, or insidiously progressive hepatitis. Not infrequently, patients with insidious AIH may develop cirrhosis and their disease activity "burns out," in which case they may become completely asymptomatic. Early after the description of AIH as a clinical entity, reported mortality was high, around 50% within 3 years of diagnosis, but the majority of these patients had an acute, symptomatic presentation. The observation that immune suppression improved the clinical course and survival of these symptomatic patients with AIH spawned the temptation to treat all patients with immunosuppressive medications to prevent the progression of liver fibrosis, with a risk of considerable morbidity from such medications. Therefore, the important question remains: Are there subsets of patients with AIH who do not require immunosuppression, either because their disease is indolent or burned out?

Before contemplating the administration of immunosuppressive agents, the physician must make a convincing diagnosis of AIH, which is often elusive. Most patients are women (80%) who present with a hepatitic pattern of liver injury. Most demonstrate serologic evidence of autoimmunity, including hypergammaglobulinemia, anti-nuclear antibodies (ANA), anti-smooth muscle antibodies (ASMA), and/or antibodies against liver-kidney microsomal antigens (anti-LKM); however, these serologic markers may be absent in up to 15% of cases. The diagnosis should include compatible liver biopsy findings, in particular, interface hepatitis, and a lymphoplasmacytic inflammatory infiltrate within the hepatic lobules. Viral serologies should be negative, and histories should rule out drug-induced hepatitis, with the recognition that certain medications can precipitate an AIH-like chronic hepatitis (eg, nitrofurantoin, diclofenac, minocycline).

After making a presumptive diagnosis of AIH, the physician must weigh the potential benefit of immunosuppression with the potential toxicity of the medications. Corticosteroids, the mainstay of the treatment of AIH, have been shown to prolong survival to more than 80% at 20 years of diagnosis but also have considerable morbidity: loss of bone mineral density, weight gain, precipitation of diabetes, hypertension, cataracts, and other complications. A steroid-sparing regimen using azathioprine (usually 1 to 1.5 mg/kg/d) in combination with a lower dose of prednisone (eg, 10 mg/d) is therefore preferred. Azathioprine, however, also has considerable toxicity, specifically, bone marrow suppression, rash, gastrointestinal intolerance, and a possible increase in the risk of developing malignancy.

Unfortunately, there are no prospective studies defining the natural history or optimal treatment of mild or inactive (burned-out) AIH. Early studies of chronic active hepatitis of various etiologies including AIH suggested that the clinical syndrome was relatively benign as long as liver biopsy showed neither cirrhosis nor bridging necrosis. However, early studies were performed before serologic markers were available to conclusively rule out viral hepatitis, and therefore these observations must be interpreted with caution. Currently, however, histologically mild AIH is generally considered a slowly progressive disease, with cirrhosis developing in fewer than 50% of patients after 15 years and with a 10-year mortality of only 10%.

Only 2 modern-era studies of asymptomatic AIH have been published in full form. In the larger study, the authors retrospectively examined the clinical courses of 31 patients with asymptomatic AIH (25% of their total cohort), which they defined as free of even nonspecific symptoms such as fatigue, arthralgias, and abdominal pain. The clinical courses of asymptomatic patients, including a subset who received immunosuppression, were compared to symptomatic patients, the vast majority of whom (90%) received immunosuppression (Table 23-1). A significant proportion of asymptomatic patients had histologic cirrhosis and would therefore fall into the "burned out AIH" category. None of the asymptomatic patients had bridging necrosis on liver biopsy. Not surprisingly, symptomatic patients had significantly higher ALT, bilirubin, IgG levels, and lobular inflammation scores compared to the asymptomatic group. Nonetheless, liver-related outcomes (transplant or death) were not significantly different in asymptomatic vs symptomatic patients. Furthermore, outcomes were not significantly different in asymptomatic patients who were, or were not, given immunosuppressive agents. Overall, 5-year and 10-year liver-related survival of symptomatic and asymptomatic patients were not significantly different, approximately 90% and 85%, respectively.

In conclusion, the prognosis of patients with untreated, asymptomatic AIH appears to be as good as treated, symptomatic AIH. The above retrospective observations suggest that there may be 2 patient populations with AIH who may not require immunosuppression: (1) asymptomatic patients with mild necroinflammatory activity on liver biopsy, and (2) those with burned-out cirrhosis. However, the same study reported that approximately 25% of asymptomatic patients eventually developed symptoms, emphasizing that such untreated patients require frequent clinical monitoring.

Table 23-1
Effect of Symptoms on Natural History and Outcome of Autoimmune Hepatitis*

	Symptomatic Presentation	*Asymptomatic Presentation*		
	(N = 94; (Treated n = 84)	All (N = 31)	Treated (n = 15)	Untreated (n = 16)
Baseline Laboratory Values				
ALT, IU/L	490	252	267	239
Bilirubin, mg/dL	8.0	1.6	1.8	1.5
IgG, mg/dL	2.81	2.1	2.1	1.8
Liver Biopsy				
Cirrhosis, %	36.2	25.8	6.7	43.8
Lobular inflammation, mean†	2.5	2.0	2.0	2.0
Endpoints				
Transplant, %	8.5	6.5	13.7	0
Liver death, %	7.4	3.2	0	6.3

*Data extracted from Feld JJ, Dinh H, Arenovich T, et al. Autoimmune hepatitis: effect of symptoms and cirrhosis on natural history and outcome. *Hepatology.* 2005;42:53-62.
†Lobular inflammation score of the Hepatic Activity Index.

Bibliography

Alvarez A, Berg A, Bianchi AB, et al. International Autoimmune Hepatitis Group report review of criteria for diagnosis of autoimmune hepatitis. *J Hepatol.* 1999;31:929-938.

Cooksley WG, Bradbear RA, Robinson W, et al. The prognosis of chronic active hepatitis without cirrhosis in relation to bridging necrosis. *Hepatology.* 1986;6:345-348.

Czaja AJ. Treatment strategies in autoimmune hepatitis. *Clin Liver Dis.* 2002;6:799-824.

Feld JJ, Dinh H, Arenovich T, et al. Autoimmune hepatitis: effect of symptoms and cirrhosis on natural history and outcome. *Hepatology.* 2005;42:53-62.

Kogan J, Safadi R, Ashur Y, et al. Prognosis of symptomatic versus asymptomatic autoimmune hepatitis: a study of 68 patients. *J Clin Gastroenterol.* 2002;35:75-81.

Sanchez-Urdazpal L, Czaja AJ, van Hoek B, et al. Prognostic features and role of liver transplantation in severe corticosteroid-treated autoimmune chronic active hepatitis. *Hepatology.* 1992;15:215.

MY PATIENT WITH AUTOIMMUNE HEPATITIS CANNOT TAKE CORTICOSTEROIDS. ARE THERE OTHER MEDICATIONS I COULD USE?

R. Todd Stravitz, MD

Widely recognized indications for the administration of immunosuppressive agents to a patient with autoimmune hepatitis (AIH) include (1) aminotransferase levels over 10-fold elevated, (2) aminotransferases over 5-fold elevated in the presence of 2-fold elevation of IgG levels, and (3) severe necroinflammatory activity on liver biopsy (bridging necrosis and/or multiascinar collapse). These indications for treatment have become doctrine after early studies documented frequent evolution to cirrhosis in such patients, and other studies demonstrated dramatic and rapid improvement with immunosuppression. Corticosteroids, either alone or in lower doses with azathioprine (1 to 1.5 mg/kg/d), are the mainstay of treatment and induce remission in 80% of such patients within 3 years of administration. However, a significant minority (15%) of patients with AIH may not be candidates for corticosteroids, including those with severe osteoporosis, poorly controlled diabetes or hypertension, steroid-induced psychosis, or those who refuse to take corticosteroids because of cosmetic concerns.

In patients with AIH who require treatment, the choice of alternatives to corticosteroids requires a superficial understanding of its immunopathogenesis. T-lymphocyte activation and proliferation constitute the primary mechanisms of hepatocellular injury in AIH (Figure 24-1). Although the hepatocyte antigens that stimulate T-lymphocytes have not been identified, the mechanisms by which T-cells become activated and proliferate are well understood. Signal I involves binding of an MHC-antigen complex to the T-cell receptor by an antigen-presenting cell (APC), triggering calcium-dependent activation of calcineurin, which dephosphorylates a cytosolic transcription factor, the nuclear factor of activated T-cells (NFAT). Dephosphorylation of NFAT induces its translocation to the nucleus and stimulation of transcription of a battery of genes

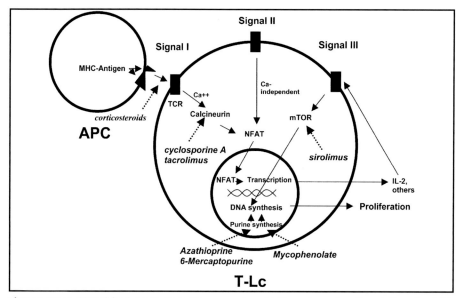

Figure 24-1. Simplified immunopathogenesis of T-lymphocyte stimulation in AIH, and sites of action of the commercially-available inhibitors of T-cell activation and proliferation. Inhibitors are indicated in italics and their sites of action are indicated with dotted arrows. APC, antigen presenting cell; IL-2, interleukin-2; MHC, major histocompatibility antigen; mTOR, mammalian target of rapamycin; NFAT, nuclear factor of activated T-cells; TCR, T-cell receptor; T-Lc, T-lymphocyte (Adapted from Vierling, JM, and Flores, PA. Evolving new therapies of autoimmune hepatitis. Clin Liver Dis. 2002; 6: 825-850, and Neuhaus, P, Klupp, J, and Langrehr, JM. mTOR inhibitors: an overview. Liver Transpl. 2001; 7: 473-484).

involved in T-cell activation, including growth factors and cytokines. Blockade of signal I appears to be pivotal to inducing remission of AIH; agents that inhibit signal I include corticosteroids and the calcineurin inhibitors, cyclosporine A (eg, Neoral®) and tacrolimus (Prograf®). Signal II is a calcium-independent pathway that enhances signal I by increasing dephosphorylation of NFAT. Oral antagonists of this costimulatory pathway are not commercially available. Signal III is generated through autocrine and paracrine stimulation of cell surface receptors by the growth factors and cytokines elaborated through signal I (most importantly, interleukin-2) and results in T-cell proliferation mediated through the mammalian target of rapamycin (mTOR). Blockade of signal III with sirolimus (also known as rapamycin; Rapamune®) inhibits T-cell progression through the cell cycle and, thus, proliferation. Other antiproliferative agents include azathioprine and its metabolite, 6-mercaptopurine (6-MP), and mycophenolate mofetil (MMF); these agents inhibit purine nucleotide, and thus DNA, biosynthesis in T-lymphocytes and other rapidly dividing cells.

A distinction should be made between medications that *induce* remission, and those that *maintain* remission, of AIH. While corticosteroids classically serve to induce remission, their use in maintaining remission is limited because of severe toxicity when administered long term. Combination therapy with medications that antagonize different sites of T-cell stimulation, therefore, may be the best strategy to minimize or avoid exposure to corticosteroids. Apart from the addition of azathioprine to cortico-

Table 24-1

Abbreviated Summary of Experience With Non-corticosteroid Medications for AIH*

Drug	N	Dose (mg/kg/d)	Levels (ng/mL)	Response
CYA[†]	30	4	250	83% BR[†]
	19	2 to 5	100 to 300	80% BR
TAC[§]	11	0.5 to 2 mg/d	3.0	91% BR
	21	6 mg/d	0.5	80% Decrease in mean ALT
MMF[‖]	8	0.5 to 3 g/d		0% BR
	5	2 g/d		71% BR KS decreased 11 to 3

*Note that most patients received the above medications because of inadequate response to, or intolerance of, corticosteroids, and many received combination therapy with corticosteroids or azathioprine.
[†] BR indicates biochemical response; CYA, cyclosporine A; KS, Knodell score; MMF, mycophenolate mofetil; TAC, tacrolimus.
[‡] Data from Alvarez et al and Malekzadeh et al.
[§] Data from Agel et al and Van Thiel et al.
[‖] Data from Czaja and Carpenter and Richardson et al.

steroids, there are no randomized, prospective studies comparing noncorticosteroid single agents or combination therapy to induce or maintain remission in AIH. Most of the available information comes from case reports or small case series of patients with AIH who did not achieve complete remission on corticosteroids. The extrapolation of results in steroid-refractory cases to patients who are corticosteroid intolerant, such as the patient presented, may not be entirely valid, since the former probably represents a group with more severe and/or recalcitrant disease. Indeed, most of the patients with steroid-refractory AIH who received other agents (Table 24-1) continued to receive various doses of corticosteroids.

In general, agents that have been reported to induce remission of AIH are those that inhibit signal I of T-cell activation. Beside corticosteroids, the calcineurin inhibitors (CNI) cyclosporine A and tacrolimus have been shown to induce biochemical remission in the majority of subjects treated for corticosteroid-refractory AIH or intolerance of corticosteroids (Table 24-1). Very few reports, however, have documented histologic improvement after administration of these agents. In addition, CNI have many adverse effects, such as hypertension, renal injury, diabetes (for tacrolimus), weight gain, hyperlipidemia (for cyclosporine), and others. Although none of the available studies in AIH have documented these toxicities, patients were generally treated with low doses for short periods and thus long-term toxicity of CNIs in AIH remains unknown. In the doses administered (Table 24-1), however, most of these reports suggest that the CNI are well tolerated in patients with AIH.

The other general class of medications used in AIH are those that maintain remission by inhibiting T-cell proliferation. The purine biosynthesis inhibitor, azathioprine, has been extensively used as a steroid-sparing agent in maintaining remission either alone or in combination with low-dose prednisone; however, azathioprine monotherapy rarely induces remission of AIH. A small case series has suggested that 6-mercaptopurine, the active metabolite of azathioprine, is also effective in maintaining remission in AIH and may be used in patients with intolerance to azathioprine because of different toxicity profiles. Finally, MMF has also been tested in patients with AIH. As with azathioprine, this purine biosynthesis inhibitor may be useful as a steroid-sparing agent to maintain remission but probably does not induce remission of AIH. Results with MMF have been mixed (Table 24-1), with one recent case series documenting very poor complete biochemical remission rates (0%), and inadequate histologic response.

As noted above, blockade of signal III might also be useful in treating patients with corticosteroid-refractory AIH or intolerance to corticosteroids by inhibiting T-cell activation and proliferation. Only 6 cases have been reported using the mTOR inhibitor, sirolimus (rapamycin), in AIH, but all of these patients were liver transplant recipients with recurrent AIH. Although disease activity was reported to improve with the addition of sirolimus to other immunosuppressive agents, extrapolation to the nontransplant population cannot be made.

In summary, the CNI appear to be useful as alternatives to corticosteroids in inducing remission in AIH. In contrast, antiproliferative agents such as azathioprine, 6-mercaptopurine, and MMF may be useful in maintaining remission in AIH. However, the available studies are extremely limited. Corticosteroid-intolerant patients with severe AIH should be considered for referral to centers with a research interest in AIH.

Bibliography

Agel BA, Machiaco V, Rosser B, et al. Efficacy of tacrolimus in the treatment of steroid refractory autoimmune hepatitis. *J Clin Gastroenterol*. 2004;38:805-809.

Alvarez F, Ciocca M, Canero-Velasco C, et al. Short-term cyclosporine induces remission of autoimmune hepatitis in children. *J Hepatol*. 1999;30:222-227.

Czaja AJ. Treatment strategies in autoimmune hepatitis. *Clin Liver Dis*. 2002;6:799-824.

Czaja AJ, Carpenter HA. Empiric therapy of autoimmune hepatitis with mycophenolate mofetil: comparison with conventional treatment for refractory disease. *J Clin Gastroenterol*. 2005;39:819-825.

Fernandez NF, Redeker AG, Vierling JM, et al. Cyclosporine therapy in patients with steroid-resistant autoimmune hepatitis. *Am J Gastroenterol*. 1999;94:241-248.

Malekzadeh R, Nasseri-Moghaddam S, Kaviani M, et al. Cyclosporine A is a promising alternative to corticosteroids in autoimmune hepatitis. *Dig Dis Sci*. 2001;46:1321-1327.

Neuhaus P, Klupp J, Langrehr JM. mTOR inhibitors: an overview. *Liver Transpl*. 2001;7:473-484.

Richardson PD, James PD, Ryder SD. Mycophenolate mofetil for maintenance of remission in autoimmune hepatitis in patients resistant or intolerant of azathioprine. *Am J Gastroenterol*. 2000;33:371-375.

Van Thiel DH, Wright H, Carroll P, et al. Tacrolimus: a potential new treatment for autoimmune chronic active hepatitis: results of an open-label preliminary trial. *Am J Gastroenterol*. 1995;90:771-776.

Vierling JM, Flores PA. Evolving new therapies of autoimmune hepatitis. *Clin Liver Dis*. 2002;6:825-850.

DO I NEED TO PERFORM A LIVER BIOPSY IN ALL PATIENTS WITH AUTOIMMUNE HEPATITIS PRIOR TO INITIATING STEROIDS?

Andres Mogollon, MD
R. Todd Stravitz, MD

Yes. Patients with suspected autoimmune hepatitis should undergo a liver biopsy before initiating corticosteroids for several reasons:

1. To establish the diagnosis of AIH. AIH can be a difficult diagnosis, and there are no noninvasively obtained data that unequivocally establish the diagnosis. In fact, an international consensus conference has published an AIH score based upon numerous clinical and laboratory parameters, including liver histology, to improve the accuracy of the diagnosis (Table 25-1). Furthermore, up to 15% of patients with AIH have negative immune serologies associated with AIH, such as anti-nuclear, anti-smooth muscle, and anti-liver/kidney microsomal antibodies; in such cases, the diagnosis of AIH virtually relies on histopathology.

2. To exclude other diseases that mimic AIH. Some liver diseases clinically resemble AIH, and distinctive histopathologic findings can discriminate these disorders from AIH (Table 25-2). For example, Wilson's disease may present as an acute hepatitis or cryptogenic cirrhosis in young patients, the age group most commonly affected by AIH. Histologically, Wilson's disease may resemble AIH, but steatohepatitis is more common, and high quantitative liver copper determination is a reliable distinguishing feature of the former. Drug-induced hepatitis may also be distinguished from AIH by a more cholestatic picture and more of an eosinophilic inflammatory infiltrate.

3. To look for evidence of variant forms of AIH (Table 25-2). AIH may occasionally coexist with features of other immune-mediated liver diseases, such as primary sclerosing cholangitis (PSC) or primary biliary cirrhosis (PBC). The treatment of AIH-PBC overlap is important to recognize, since ursodiol is commonly recommended in addition to corticosteroids.

Table 25-1

Histologic Features of the International AIH Scoring System*†

Histologic Features	*Points*
Interface hepatitis (piecemeal necrosis)	+3
Plasma cell inflammatory infiltrate	+1
Regenerating hepatocyte aggregates (rosettes)	+1
None of above	−5
Biliary changes suggestive of PBC or PSC	−3
Other prominent histologic features suggestive of a different etiology	−3

*Other clinical features account for a maximum of 7 points and laboratory features account for 14 points. Patients with >15 points have definite AIH and those with 10 to 15 points have "probable" AIH.
† Modified from Alvarez et al.

Table 25-2

Differential Diagnosis of AIH by Liver Biopsy Features

Diagnosis	*Prominent Histologic Features*
AIH (classical)	Interface hepatitis (piecemeal necrosis), lymphocytic inflammatory infiltrate with plasma cells, lobular hepatitis
Wilson's disease	Steatosis > interface hepatitis/piecemeal necrosis; elevated quantitative copper
Non-alcoholic fatty liver disease	Macrovesicular steatosis, PMN-predominant inflammatory infiltrate, Mallory bodies, ballooning degeneration of hepatocytes, sinusoidal fibrosis
Drug hepatitis	Cholestasis or mixed cholestatic/hepatitic pattern of injury, prominent eosinophilic inflammatory infiltrate
AIH/PBC overlap	AIH features, with prominent lymphocytic portal inflammation and bile duct injury; cholestasis
AIH/PSC overlap	AIH features, with fibrous obliteration of bile ducts; cholestasis; bile duct proliferation

Modified from Carpenter HA, Czaja AJ. The role of histologic evaluation in the diagnosis and management of autoimmune hepatitis and its variants. *Clin Liver Dis*. 2002;6:685-705

4. To assess the need for immunosuppression. The treatment of AIH with corticosteroids carries significant morbidity, including loss of bone mineral density, steroid-induced hypertension, weight gain, diabetes, cosmetic changes, cataracts, and mood alterations, among others. Some patients with mild histologic changes of AIH (for example, mild inflammation and piecemeal necrosis) may not require corticosteroids, since they have a good prognosis untreated. In contrast, severe histopathology in a patient with AIH is an absolute indication for corticosteroid administration, since the findings of bridging necrosis or mutlilobular collapse have been associated with rapid progression to cirrhosis. Although the degree of aminotransferase and gamma-globulin elevation generally correlates to the severity of histologic abnormalities, they are not reliable markers of these findings.

5. To document a baseline for posttreatment comparison. Treatment of AIH with corticosteroids typically normalizes transaminases, so-called biochemical remission. However, biochemical remission does not guarantee histologic remission, and therefore a baseline histology before corticosteroid treatment will help guide the decision regarding discontinuation of treatment. In addition, approximately 15% of patients do not normalize aminotransferases with immunosuppression, in which case the physician should consider re-biopsy to compare to pretreatment histology. This assessment will help guide a decision to initiate more aggressive immunosuppression in such incomplete responders.

6. To estimate prognosis. The finding of cirrhosis on pretreatment liver biopsy is a poor prognostic sign for death or the eventual need for liver transplantation (relative risk of 6.79 in one study). Even patients with completely asymptomatic AIH may have cirrhosis on their index liver biopsy. Biopsy at presentation therefore determines prognosis: bridging fibrosis predicts development of cirrhosis and cirrhosis predicts a lower 5-year to 10-year survival.

Bibliography

Alvarez F, Berg PA, Bianchi FB, et al. International Autoimmune Hepatitis Group report: review of criteria for diagnosis of autoimmune hepatitis. *J Hepatol.* 1999;31:929-938.

Carpenter HA, Czaja AJ. The role of histologic evaluation in the diagnosis and management of autoimmune hepatitis and its variants. *Clin Liver Dis.* 2002;6:685-705.

Feld JJ, Dinh H, et al. Autoimmune hepatitis: effect of symptoms and cirrhosis on natural history and outcome. *Hepatology.* 2005;42:53-62.

SECTION V

FATTY LIVER DISEASE

WHICH PATIENTS WITH FATTY LIVER DISEASE ON ULTRASOUND REQUIRE A LIVER BIOPSY?

Arun J. Sanyal, MD
B. Marie Reid, MD

Over two-thirds of the general population of the United States is either overweight or obese. Obesity and the metabolic syndrome are the most common risk factors for the development of nonalcoholic fatty liver disease (NAFLD). Indeed, NAFLD is considered to be the hepatic manifestation of the metabolic syndrome. The clinical-histologic spectrum of NAFLD extends from a nonalcoholic fatty liver (NAFL) to nonalcoholic steatohepatitis (NASH). NASH can progress to cirrhosis in up to 15% to 20% of subjects. It is generally estimated that about 30% of the US population has NAFLD and that 3% to 4% of individuals have NASH. Given the commonality of these conditions, the clinician is frequently confronted with a situation when an abdominal ultrasound performed for unrelated conditions or abnormal liver enzymes demonstrates an echogenic liver, which is often interpreted as evidence of fatty liver disease. The key question in such cases is should a liver biopsy be performed?

Can a Liver Ultrasound Diagnose a Fatty Liver Accurately?[1]

The characteristics of a fatty liver include a hyperechoic liver where the echo-texture of the liver is brighter than the kidney and blurring of vascular margins. These are relatively sensitive but nonspecific findings and can also be seen in many other causes of chronic liver disease. They do not provide any distinction between steatosis and steatohepatitis and, in the absence of ascites and overt findings of portal hypertension, provides no information on the stage of the disease. It is, however, the least expensive of the imaging modalities available for evaluation of fatty liver disease and is therefore commonly used.

The specificity for the diagnosis of hepatic steatosis can be improved with a computed tomography (CT) scan or magnetic resonance imaging (MRI) but with an exponential increase in the cost of the procedure. Also, neither a CT scan nor an MRI can distinguish between NAFL and NASH and have the same limitations with respect to fibrosis as an ultrasound.

What Information Can Be Obtained From a Liver Biopsy?

As with any procedure, before performing a liver biopsy, one must consider the information that will be obtained from it, the importance of this information for patient management, the risks involved, and the cost of the procedure. A liver biopsy provides 3 key pieces of information with respect to fatty liver disease: (a) it definitively allows one to exclude alternate causes of elevated liver enzymes, (b) it is the only method to distinguish NAFL from NASH with certainty, and (c) it provides information on the stage of the disease (ie, the degree of fibrosis).

Risks of a Liver Biopsy

A liver biopsy is generally well tolerated. There are, however, certain unavoidable risks and potential complications. The most common complication is pain at the biopsy site and referred pain at the right shoulder. Rarely, other more serious complications such as pneumothorax, hemothorax, and bile peritonitis occur, requiring more intensive monitoring and evaluation. At the Mayo clinic, 9212 liver biopsies were performed with data prospectively recorded to identify risk factors for major bleeding. There were 10 fatal and 22 nonfatal hemorrhages (0.11% and 0.24%, respectively). When compared to those patients who did not experience a hemorrhage, malignancy, age, sex, and the number of passes were the only predictable risk factors for an adverse event.[2]

Approach to Subject With an Echogenic Liver[3]

The need for a liver biopsy is often dictated by the clinical scenario in which the sonographic findings are discovered. In subjects with elevated liver enzymes, it is imperative to first exclude other common causes of liver enzyme elevation and to obtain a good history with respect to alcohol consumption. Subjects who consume more than 2 or 3 alcoholic beverages daily or those who binge drink (eg, a 6-pack of beer on the weekend) should be counseled to stop drinking and should be reassessed after at least 3 months of abstinence. In subjects with persistently elevated liver enzymes, it is known that 25% to 30% of subjects do not have NAFLD. In fact, 5% to 7% of such cases have normal liver histology. Given the frequent coexistence of NAFLD and features of the metabolic syndrome, it appears logical that if such features are present, then the likelihood of having fatty liver disease is higher. Conversely, if such features are absent, ie, a normal body mass index and absence of hypertension, diabetes or dyslipidemia, the probability of having an

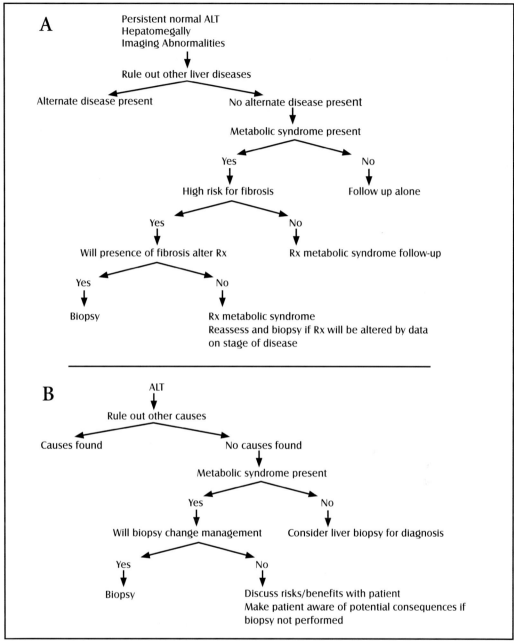

Figure 26-1. (A) An algorithm for diagnosis in patients with persistent normal liver enzymes who present with either hepatomegaly or imaging abnormalities. (B) An algorithm for diagnosis in patients with elevated liver enzymes.

alternate diagnosis rises. It must be remembered that this is not an "absolute" method for identification of subjects with NAFLD. Figure 26-1 outlines an example of a cost effective algorithm in the evaluation of the clinical significance of LFTs.

In some cases, where a diagnostic dilemma is present or where demonstration of normal histology or mild nonspecific findings will allow an individual to get life insurance, the benefits and potential risks should be discussed and a biopsy performed if the benefits are considered to outweigh the risks.

In subjects with the metabolic syndrome, it is often argued that knowing whether NASH is present is not useful in the absence of approved treatment for NASH. This is an evolving field and numerous studies have now demonstrated the benefits of weight-loss surgery on NAFLD. Also, emerging data indicate that thiazolidinediones may also be effective therapy, although they are associated with weight gain and occasional heart failure. Thus, in subjects where demonstration of advanced histology may push one toward bariatric surgery, enrollment in a clinical trial or off-label use of pharmacologic agents associated with side effects, a liver biopsy is mandatory. The odds of identification of such individuals are vastly improved by focusing on those who are over 50 years of age, extremely obese, and have other features of the metabolic syndrome especially diabetes.[4,5] Once again, these are not absolute criteria and the potential likelihood of having aggressive disease (NASH with cytologic ballooning and/or bridging fibrosis) is increased with the coexistance of other features of the metabolic syndrome.

In some individuals with a high risk of having advanced disease, there is value to knowing whether it has progressed to cirrhosis or if bridging fibrosis is present. In the latter instance, this knowledge provides an opportunity to intervene by pharmacologic methods, mainly by clinical trials, and by bariatric surgery. In those with cirrhosis, the risk of developing hepatocellular cancer is about 10% over a 10-year time frame and a screening regimen with serial sonograms and alpha-fetoproteins should be instituted. Such patients should also undergo screening endoscopy to look for varices and have to be followed closely. Once again, increasing age, severity of obesity, particularly abdominal obesity, and the presence of additional features of the metabolic syndrome are important markers of advanced disease and useful to identify those who need a biopsy.

In summary, the indications for a liver biopsy in those with an echogenic liver are:

- Persistent elevation of liver enzymes despite attempts to improve weight by diet and exercise
- Those over 50 years of age with multiple features of the metabolic syndrome, eg, obesity and diabetes or hypertension

An individualized decision has to be made in all other cases based on what clinical information is likely to be obtained from the biopsy, how it will affect management and the cost of the procedure.

References

1. Saadeh S, Younossi ZM, Remer EM, et al. The utility of radiological imaging in nonalcoholic fatty liver disease. *Gastroenterology.* 2002;123:745-750.
2. McGill DB, Rakela J, Zinsmeister AR, Ott BJA. 21-Year experience with major hemorrhage after percutaneous liver biopsy. *Gastroenterology.* 1990;99:1396-1400.
3. Ramesh S, Sanyal AJ. Evaluation and management of non-alcoholic steatohepatitis. *J Hepatol.* 2005;42(suppl 1:S2-S12.
4. Angulo P, Keach JC, Batts KP, Lindor KD. Independent predictors of liver fibrosis in patients with nonalcoholic steatohepatitis. *Hepatology.* 1999;30:1356-1362.
5. Dixon JB, Bhathal PS, O'Brien PE. Nonalcoholic fatty liver disease: predictors of nonalcoholic steatohepatitis and liver fibrosis in the severely obese. *Gastroenterology.* 2001;121:91-100.

AN OBESE PATIENT WITH HYPERCHOLESTEROLEMIA WAS RECENTLY STARTED ON A STATIN AND IS NOW FOUND TO HAVE ELEVATED SERUM LIVER TRANSAMINASES. DO I NEED TO STOP THIS MEDICATION?

Arun J. Sanyal, MD
Jayanta Choudhury, MD

Dyslipidemia is a common risk factor associated with both nonalcoholic fatty liver disease (NAFLD) and cardiovascular disease. It is also well known that the metabolic syndrome is almost universally present in NAFLD and dyslipidemia forms an important modifiable part of this condition. The modification of dyslipidemia with statins or 3-hydroxy-3-methylglutaryl-coenzyme A reductase inhibitors (HMGCoA) is common in clinical practice and an increasing number of people are being placed on these medications. Hence, it is not uncommon to have patients with the metabolic syndrome and dyslipidemia being started on statins and subsequently detected to have abnormal liver enzymes during routine follow-up. As one of the well-known adverse effects of statins is abnormal liver enzymes, the detection of the same in this population of patients raises an important therapeutic dilemma; ie, should the statins be stopped?

Statins and Transaminase Elevation

The association of elevation of liver enzymes and the use of a statin group of medication has been consistently seen across all the relevant studies that have been done with these medications.[1] It is currently estimated that the elevation of aminotransferases >3 times the upper limit of normal occurs in <1% of patients that are placed on these medications.[2] The incidence of elevation is somewhat higher when combination therapy of two antilipidemic drugs such as ezetimibe and statin or larger doses of drugs such as atorvastatin are used. It is also well known that spontaneous fluctuation of transaminases occurs over time in the population. Similar fluctuations are also seen in patients with dyslipidemia who have been treated with placebo in studies looking at the effects of statins on liver function. The whole situation is further confounded by the presence of concomitant NAFLD in a large percentage of the same cohort of patients as well as the consumption of other non-statin medications and/or alcohol.

Statins and Acute Liver Failure

The significance of elevated liver enzymes with normal bilirubin levels is not entirely clear. There is currently no evidence to suggest that isolated elevation of transaminases in patients who are placed on statins leads to either acute or chronic liver injury. Liver failure secondary to statin therapy has been reported but is extremely rare and is thought mainly due to an idiosyncratic drug effect. Review of liver transplant data over a period of 12 years (1990 to 2002) has shown that out of 51 741 liver transplants, only 3 patients had acute liver failure that was attributed to statins.[3] It is estimated that the incidence of true statin-induced liver failure is as low as 1 per million person/years of use.[4] In some subjects with statin-induced acute liver failure, clinical features of autoimmune hepatitis develop, including a positive anti-nuclear antibody. Once again, this is rare. Hence the overall consensus among hepatologist is that liver failure requiring liver transplant may rarely occur with statin therapy but the risk is remote and should not preclude their use.

Statins and Chronic Liver Disease/Cirrhosis

The use of medications that are metabolized by the liver in patients who have either chronic liver diseases or compensated Child's A cirrhosis is a common concern of patients as well as physicians taking care of these individuals. The recommendations of the Liver Task Force advising the National Lipid Association are that both chronic liver disease and compensated cirrhosis are not contraindications for statin therapy.[2] The pharmacokinetics of statins in compensated cirrhotics and chronic liver disease is unaltered and the incidence of elevation of liver enzymes due to statin therapy in this group of patients is same as the general population. Decompensated cirrhosis is a potentially fatal condition unless transplanted and the value of statin therapy in such patients is debatable. Similar recommendations hold for patients with either acute or subacute liver failure due to the limited role that lipid lowering has in these potentially life-threatening scenarios.

Statins and Nonalcoholic Fatty Liver Disease

The prevalence of obesity in the population and the awareness among health care professionals about nonalcoholic fatty liver disease has increased over the past few decades.

As the diagnosis of NAFLD is often incidental and the disease itself asymptomatic, the true prevalence of this condition has been underreported, despite the fact that the risk factors associated with the metabolic syndrome and NAFLD are largely the same as that associated with cardiovascular disease and have been targeted by interventions such as statin therapy over the past several decades. Hence, it is more than likely that patients receiving statin therapy for cardiac risk modifications have underlying NAFLD. Despite the decades of use of these drugs in this population, there is no evidence of increased incidence of advanced liver disease in this population. Moreover, in large studies like the Dallas Heart Study, it was seen that compared to placebo, statin use was not associated with either greater frequency of hepatic steatosis (38% vs 34%) or increased serum transaminases (15% vs 13%).[5] In addition, it was seen that statin use was not associated with increased transaminases in patients who had preexisting hepatic steatosis.

Because hepatic steatosis is present in >80% of patients with dyslipidemia and abnormal liver enzymes, aggressive measures to lower the lipid levels with drugs may be an attractive option in management of patients with fatty liver disease. However, it still remains to be proven whether lowering serum lipid levels actually alters hepatic fat content and reverses changes associated with steatohepatitis. There has been no evidence to date that patients with abnormal liver enzymes secondary to fatty liver disease are at increased risk of statin-induced liver toxicity compared to their normal liver enzymes counterparts.

Statins and Surveillance of Liver Function

The surveillance of liver enzymes in patients who are taking statins and management of occasional abnormal liver enzymes that are detected as a consequence is another area of concern among physicians. Many hepatologists dealing with these patients feel that monitoring of liver enzymes is unnecessary in patients receiving statin therapy because severe statin toxicity is likely idiosyncratic and no data exist to show that this form of surveillance actually helps to identify those patients. Moreover, it is felt that presence of abnormal enzymes detected in patients who otherwise may benefit from statin therapy may lead to discontinuation of statins. This may lead to inadequate correction of a potentially reversible risk factor associated with cardiovascular-related as well as possibly liver-related morbidity and mortality. There are other additional concerns with regard to overall costs and patient anxiety regarding periodic liver enzymes monitoring while on statin therapy.

An Approach to the Subject on Statins Who Develops Elevated Liver Enzymes

A full hepatic panel and measures of hepatic synthetic functions are indicated in the subject on statins who develops elevated liver enzymes. In addition, the subject should be evaluated clinically. All potentially hepatotoxic drugs should be stopped if the aspartate aminotransferase (AST) and alanine aminotrasferase (ALT) are more than 10-fold elevated or if there is any evidence of hepatic synthetic dysfunction; ie, elevation of conjugated bilirubin or prolongation of prothrombin time. Also, it is important to exclude other common causes of acute liver injury; eg, viral hepatitis.

For lesser degrees of liver enzyme elevation and normal bilirubin and prothrombin time, the likelihood of development of severe liver toxicity is low. Such patients can be followed up with repeat measurements of liver enzymes within a week or 2 and then at 3-month to 6-month intervals. The early time points provide data on the likelihood of acute liver failure while subjects with persistent elevations should be evaluated for chronic liver disease, especially nonalcoholic fatty liver disease. Statins do not need to be discontinued in subjects with this degree of liver enzyme elevation. Once again, it is important to perform a thorough clinical exam and exclude other common causes of liver diseases.

Finally, if either statin-induced liver toxicity is diagnosed or cannot be excluded in the setting of abnormal liver function tests, it is recommended that statin not be restarted and alternative antihyperlipidemic therapy should be considered.

References

1. Chalasani N. Statins and hepatotoxicity: focus on patients with fatty liver. *Hepatology.* 2005;41:690-695.
2. Cohen DE, Anania FA, Chalasani N. An assessment of statin safety by hepatologists. *Am J Cardiol.* 2006;97:77C-81C.
3. Russo MW, Galanko JA, Shrestha R, Fried MW, Watkins P. Liver transplantation for acute liver failure from drug induced liver injury in the United States. *Liver Transpl.* 2004;10:1018-1023.
4. Law M, Rudnicka AR. Statin safety: a systematic review. *Am J Cardiol.* 2006;97:52C-60C.
5. Browning JD. Statins and hepatic steatosis: perspectives from the Dallas Heart Study. *Hepatology.* 2006;44:466-471.

WHAT IS THE BEST TREATMENT TO UTILIZE IN A PATIENT WITH FATTY LIVER DISEASE AND TYPE 2 DIABETES MELLITUS?

Arun J. Sanyal, MD
Puneet Puri, MD

Nonalcoholic fatty liver disease (NAFLD) is a common cause of chronic liver disease in the United States.[1] NAFLD includes a nonalcoholic fatty liver (NAFL) and nonalcoholic steatohepatitis (NASH). NASH can progress to cirrhosis in up to 15% of subjects. NAFLD is associated with abdominal obesity, type 2 diabetes, hypertension, and dyslipidemia, together known as the *metabolic syndrome*, which is characterized by the presence of insulin resistance. The main focus of management is to treat the risk factors for NAFLD. The presence of obesity and T2DM independently influences the severity of liver disease. Therefore, therapeutic intervention in NAFLD deserves special attention.

Weight Management

Lifestyle modifications and pharmacotherapy usually result in short-term modest weight loss and may substantially improve the metabolic profile. The successful principles of weight management include ~10% weight reduction from baseline at about 1 to 2 pounds/week followed by maintenance. A daily deficit of 500 to 1000 calories and about 150 min/week of moderate-intensity aerobic physical activity is recommended to achieve above goals.[2,3] For diabetic individuals, the American Diabetes Association guidelines for diet should be followed. Pharmacologic agents can augment lifestyle modifications in weight loss. The currently approved drugs orlistat and sibutramine are available options in subjects with BMI > 30 kg/m^2 or BMI > 27 kg/m^2 associated with comorbidities; eg, T2DM, sleep apnea.[2] Rimonabant, a selective cannabinoid-1 receptor blocker at 20 mg/d, in combination with diet and exercise, was shown to significantly reduce body weight and improve several metabolic risk factors in multiple trials.[4] However, its efficacy in NAFLD and its overall long-term benefits need to be evaluated.

SURGICAL OPTION (TABLE 28-1)

Bariatric surgery is the most effective therapy for severe obesity and significantly improves morbidity and mortality. It is indicated for those with BMI > 40 or BMI ≥ 35 kg/m^2 with comorbid conditions.[5] Different techniques include:

1. Malabsorptive procedures

    a. Jejunoileal bypass (JIB): This involves an intestinal anastomosis proximal to the ileocecal valve. Nearly 70% of subjects attained sustained weight loss but had high incidence of complications. Importantly, 10% of subjects developed liver failure during a 15-year follow-up. This is no longer recommended as a weight-loss procedure.

    b. Biliopancreatic diversion with duodenal switch (BPD-DS): Primarily malabsorptive, it is improvised JIB and modified BPD with lower incidence of liver disease. It is more effective in and should be reserved for those with BMI > 50 kg/m^2.

2. Restrictive procedures

    a. Vertical band gastroplasty (VBG): This is performed with a circumferential band placed around gastric pouch created by stapling the gastric fundus. A less favorable weight loss and adverse effects limit its widespread use.

    b. Laparoscopic adjustable gastric banding (LAGB): Low morbidity and mortality without altering the anatomy make LAGB an attractive option. The US experience is encouraging for acceptable weight loss and modest resolution of comorbidities.

3. Combination of malabsorptive and restrictive procedure

    a. Roux-en Y gastric bypass (RYGBP): This is the gold standard for bariatric surgery, with excellent outcomes and low morbidity. The RYGBP is constructed using a 15-mL to 20-mL gastric pouch and Roux-en Y gastrojejunostomy. The laparoscopic approach to RYGBP produces comparable and sustained weight loss with improvement in comorbidities.

The available data suggest significantly improved steatosis, necroinflammatory activity, and hepatic fibrosis following bariatric surgery. This is accompanied by marked improvement in T2DM and insulin sensitivity. However, the long-term outcome of bariatric surgery in patients with morbid obesity and NAFLD is unknown. Although there are no studies to compare RYGBP, BPD-DS, LABP, and VBG in NAFLD, transient AST/ALT elevation in BPD-DS and worsening fibrosis in a subset of patients with VBG were noted.[6,7] The presence of cirrhosis may have adverse outcome and therefore patients should be carefully selected.

Pharmacologic Treatment of NASH

There is currently no clearly defined pharmacologic treatment for NAFLD. Metformin, a biguanide, activates AMP kinase, primarily reducing hepatic glucose production, but also decreases lipid synthesis and increases lipid oxidation. Although metformin improved

Table 28-1

Summary of Different Types of Weight-Loss Surgeries*

Parameter	RYGBP	BPD-DS	VBG	LAGB
Weight Loss				
% EBW	65 to 70	~70	50 to 60	50
% BMI		~35	25 to 30	25
NAFLD	Significantly improves	Significantly improves	Significantly improves except fibrosis, may get worse	Significantly improves
Diabetes	Significantly improves or resolves 65% to 95%	Significantly improves or resolves 65% to 95%	Improves or resolves	Improves or resolves 40% to 65%
Operative				
Mortality	0.5% to 1.0%	1%	0.1%	0.1%
Morbidity	5%	5%	5%	5%
Complication	Stomach dilation, ventral hernia	Malabsorption Increased transaminases, resolve after 6 months	Food/pill impaction Outlet absorption	Gastric prolapse, stomal obstruction, pouch dilation
Type	Restrictive/ malabsorptive	Malabsorptive/ restrictive	Restrictive	Restrictive
Use in the United States	87%	2%	1.4%	9%

*EBW indicates excess body weight; BMI, body mass index; NAFLD, nonalcoholic fatty liver disease; RYGBP, roux-en Y gastric bypass; BPD-DS, biliopancreatic diversion with duodenal switch; VBG, vertical band gastroplasty; LAGB, laparoscopic adjustable gastric banding.

hepatic steatosis and inflammation in animal models, this has not been corroborated in human studies despite a decrease in ALT and liver size.

Thiazolidinediones, eg, roziglitazone and pioglitazone, act via peroxisome proliferator activating receptor and improve insulin sensitivity. Previous trials with thiazolidinediones showed metabolic and histologic improvement in NASH.[8] Caution should, however, be exercised while interpreting these data due to the small number of subjects. A clear picture should hopefully emerge from a large NIH-sponsored PIVENS clinical trial. Given the potential risk for hepatotoxicity with these drugs, the patients should be carefully monitored. Regarding insulin therapy in subjects with T2DM and NAFLD, there are no prospective data. NAFLD, however, should not be a contraindication for insulin treatment in T2DM, if indicated. Incretins are currently being investigated in the treatment of T2DM.

In two small prospective studies, pentoxifylline, a TNF-α inhibitor, improved the clinical, biochemical, and metabolic parameters in subjects with NASH. However, large randomized control trials to evaluate histologic improvement and safety are needed. Encouraging results from RIO trials merit evaluation of rimonabant, the selective cannabinoid-1 receptor blocker, in the treatment of NAFLD. Several other agents, including lipid-lowering medications (statins, fibrates, and omega-3 fatty acids), antioxidants (vitamins E and C), cytoprotective therapies (ursodeoxycholic acid; betaine,a precursor of s-adenosyl methionine), and losartan, for the prevention of fibrosis have been studied in NASH with variable results and remain experimental.

Approach to the Patient (Figure 28-1)

There are currently no data to support evidence-based recommendations for the management of NAFLD in T2DM. The recommendations below should therefore be considered to be expert opinion only. It is our approach to use the BMI as a guide for therapy. The underlying principle is to try to find treatment that will benefit both NAFLD and T2DM. Subjects with a BMI > 35 clearly improve their diabetes and many subjects no longer require anti-diabetic drugs after bariatric surgery. For those with a BMI between 35 and 40, we recommend an adjustable band gastroplasty. On the other hand, it is our experience that the response is both better and more durable with a Roux-en Y proximal gastric bypass in those with a BMI > 40. There are now numerous studies demonstrating improvement in NASH and even hepatic fibrosis after these operations.

For subjects with a BMI < 35, the aggressiveness with which we approach therapy is determined by the liver histology. In those with mild histologic changes, ie, fatty liver or fatty liver with inflammation only, we recommend optimization of diabetes control along with diet and exercise. In subjects with aggressive histology (cytologic ballooning along with inflammation and steatosis; advanced fibrosis), we additionally consider pharmacologic treatment. Thiazolidinediones are our first-line drugs in subjects with T2DM and NASH and are preferred over metformin. Also, regardless of the liver histology, those who need pharmacologic treatment for their T2DM should receive a thiazolidinedione. Alternatively, subjects with T2DM and aggressive NASH may be referred to a tertiary care center for enrollment in a clinical trial. Pharmacologic agents for weight management may be used in this population if indicated based on published guidelines.

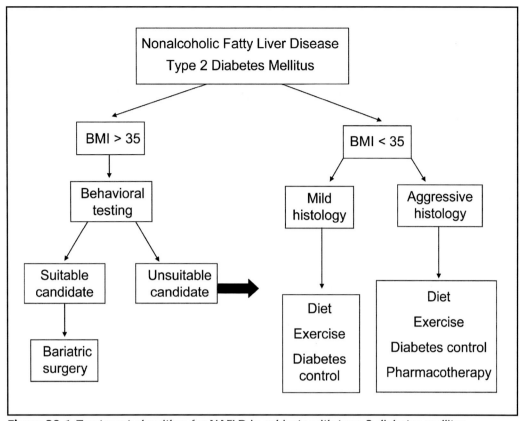

Figure 28-1. Treatment algorithm for NAFLD in subjects with type 2 diabetes mellitus.

References

1. Sanyal AJ. AGA technical review on nonalcoholic fatty liver disease. *Gastroenterology.* 2002;123:1705-1725.-
2. Kiernan M, Winkleby MA. Identifying patients for weight-loss treatment: an empirical evaluation of the NHLBI obesity education initiative expert panel treatment recommendations. *Arch Intern Med.* 2000;160:2169-2176.
3. Zivkovik AM, German JB, Sanyal AJ. Comparative review of diets for metabolic syndrome: implications for nonalcoholic fatty liver disease. *Am J Clin Nutr.* In press.
4. Hollander P. Endocannabinoid blockade for improving glycemic control and lipids in patients with type 2 diabetes mellitus. *Am J Med.* 2007;120:S18-S28.
5. Buchwald H. Consensus conference statement bariatric surgery for morbid obesity: health implications for patients, health professionals, and third-party payers. *Surg Obes Relat Dis.* 2005;3:371-381.
6. Keshishian A, Zahriya K, Willes EB. Duodenal switch has no detrimental effects on hepatic function and improves hepatic steatohepatitis after 6 months. *Obes Surg.* 2005;15:1418-1423.
7. Stratopoulos C, Papakonstantinou A, Terzis I, et al. Changes in liver histology accompanying massive weight loss after gastroplasty for morbid obesity. *Obes Surg.* 2005;15:1154-1160.
8. Belfort R, Harrison SA, Brown K, et al. A placebo-controlled trial of pioglitazone in subjects with nonalcoholic steatohepatitis. *N Engl J Med.* 2006;355:2297-2307.

MY PATIENT WITH CHRONIC HEPATITIS C ALSO HAS EVIDENCE OF NONALCOHOLIC STEATOHEPATITIS ON HIS LIVER BIOPSY. WHAT CAN I DO TO INCREASE HIS CHANCE OF RESPONDING TO PEGINTERFERON AND RIBAVIRIN TREATMENT?

Arun J. Sanyal, MD
Onpang Cheung, MD, MPH

HCV and Steatosis

Hepatitis C virus (HCV) is one of the most common causes of chronic liver disease, affecting 130 million individuals worldwide and approximately 2.7 million Americans. Twenty percent of these patients will potentially progress to cirrhosis. Nonspecific histologic features of steatosis and Mallory body–like material within hepatocytes are seen in 30% to 70% of patients with chronic hepatitis C (CHC) and are thought to be related to both viral (HCV genotype 3) and host factors (conditions associated with the metabolic syndrome). Genotype 3 HCV directly produces hepatic steatosis by interfering with hepatic triglyceride secretion and resolution of steatosis is observed with loss of viremia after antiviral treatment.[1] Genotype 3 is the only subtype that has been shown to correlate with a higher grade of steatosis in patients with CHC independent of other host-related factors; ie, nonalcoholic fatty liver disease (NAFLD).[2] The steatosis noted in subjects with genotype 1 HCV, on the other hand, is associated with obesity and insulin resistance. HCV core proteins have been implicated in the pathogenesis of hepatic steatosis. Moreover, impairment of intracellular insulin signaling by modulation of the cytokine-sensitive c-jun N terminal kinase is an important mechanism contributing to hepatitis C in genotype 1–infected subjects.

NAFLD/NASH Superimposed With HCV

NAFLD is the most common cause of chronic liver disease in the world, affecting up to 30% of the general population. Its spectrum of histologic changes ranges from simple steatosis to nonalcoholic steatohepatitis (NASH), which can progress to cirrhosis in 15% to 20% of patients. The histological diagnosis of NASH is made by the presence of pericentral steatosis, cytologic ballooning, neutrophilic and lymphocytic intralobular infiltration, and variable degree of pericellular fibrosis in zone 3. NAFLD is now considered the hepatic manifestation of the metabolic syndrome and is strongly associated with insulin resistance and obesity.

The presence of NAFLD in a subject with hepatitis C is most often inferred from the presence of macrovesicular steatosis. The diagnosis of NASH is often difficult because hepatitis C can cause both lobular and portal inflammation. This diagnosis is usually made when, in addition to findings of hepatitis C, ie, lobular and portal inflammation and portal-based fibrosis, there is steatosis, cytologic ballooning, pericentral perisinusoidal fibrosis, and Mallory hyaline. It must be remembered that concomitant alcohol abuse can cause these findings also, especially in the population of subjects with hepatitis C.

Impact of Concomitant NAFLD on Liver Disease and Virologic Response in HCV-Infected Subjects

The presence of concomitant NAFLD with HCV is associated with a higher degree of fibrosis in cross-sectional studies.[3] The fibrosis is most marked when cytologic ballooning is present along with steatosis.[4] This has been linked to the features of insulin resistance. Hyperinsulinemia, a key feature of insulin resistance, has been shown to increase collagen production by hepatic stellate cells. Also, hyperleptinemia associated with the insulin-resistant state increases collagen production by hepatic stellate cells.

Current standard HCV treatment includes a combination of pegylated interferon-alfa (IFN-α) and ribavirin with a sustained virologic response rate (SVR) of 54% to 63%. Generally, HCV genotype 2 and 3 are more likely to achieve SVR than genotype 1. Factors that have been shown to influence therapy response include age, duration of infection, HCV genotypes, gender, race, HLA type, viral burden, alcohol consumption, hepatic steatosis and cirrhosis, and obesity. Hepatic steatosis is an independent risk factor for failure to achieve virologic response. This failure is further worsened by the concomitant presence of cytologic ballooning, a feature of steatohepatitis that may coexist with hepatitis C.

Recommendations to Increase the Efficacy of Antiviral Therapy for CHC Patients With Concurrent NASH

Subjects with genotype 2 and 3 infections have a high probability of sustained virologic response regardless of the presence of hepatic steatosis. In such subjects, one does not necessarily need to treat the NASH before proceeding to therapy of HCV. On the other hand, subjects with genotype 1 infection should be evaluated for their risk of becoming a virologic nonresponder. Two approaches can be taken in those at high risk: (1) modify HCV treatment to increase the response rate and (2) treat NASH as a way to improve virologic response.

It is critically important to start with an adequate dosage of both pegylated interferon and ribavirin. The patients must be educated about the side effect profile of therapy and support should be provided to help them cope with these. This is vitally important to ensure compliance with therapy, a key factor that determines virologic response. This author recommends checking the HCV virus count after 4 weeks of therapy to learn whether an early virologic response is present. If present, such patients are highly likely to respond. Whether treatment should be prolonged to 18 months in subjects who have a late virologic response at 3 months is controversial. The likelihood of sustained virologic response drops exponentially if the virus count has not become undetectable after 3 months of therapy.

It must be noted that, while the presence of concomitant NAFLD increases the risk of failure to clear the virus with first-line treatment, there are no data on the value of treating NAFLD as a way to improve virologic response. Despite this lack of data, there is considerable enthusiasm to tackle NAFLD as a modifiable risk factor to optimize the response to antiviral therapy in subjects with HCV.

The optimal treatment for any condition is one that is rational, effective, safe, easy to provide, and relatively inexpensive. To date, optimal therapy for NAFLD remains to be defined. The focus of treatment is therefore to treat the underlying risk factors, ie, obesity and insulin resistance, or to protect the liver with hepato-protectants. Improvement of obesity and insulin resistance is a laudable therapeutic goal simply on the basis of the improvement of cardiovascular risks that ensue. It is therefore reasonable to treat obesity when present. In the absence of any data on the utility of treating NASH to improve virologic response, it is this author's approach not to withhold antiviral therapy but to institute a diet and lifestyle plan shortly prior to starting treatment. In subjects in whom a virologic response is most urgently required, ie, those with aggressive inflammation and/or bridging fibrosis, it may be reasonable to aggressively treat the obesity with the goal of improving insulin resistance and thus the fatty liver. There are several excellent reviews on the approach to weight management and the reader is referred to these for a detailed discussion of the subject.[5,6] Emerging data suggest that thiazolidinediones, eg, pioglitazone may be effective in improving steatohepatitis. In the absence of large-scale studies clearly defining the value of such agents for NASH, their use should be restricted to those with aggressive steatohepatitic changes, especially if they are diabetic.

References

1. Castera L, et al. Effect of antiviral treatment on evolution of liver steatosis in patients with chronic hepatitis C: indirect evidence of a role of hepatitis C virus genotype 3 in steatosis. *Gut.* 2004;53:420-424.
2. Rubbia-Brandt L, et al. Steatosis affects chronic hepatitis C progression in a genotype specific way. *Gut.* 2004;53:406-412.
3. Ong JP, et al. Chronic hepatitis C and superimposed nonalcoholic fatty liver disease. *Liver.* 2001;21:266-271.
4. Sanyal AJ, et al. Nonalcoholic fatty liver disease in patients with hepatitis C is associated with features of the metabolic syndrome. *Am J Gastroenterol.* 2003;98:2064-2071.
5. Zivkovic AM, JBG, Sanyal AJ. Comparative review of diets for metabolic syndrome: implications for nonalcoholic fatty liver disease. *Am J Clin Nutr.* In press.
6. National Heart Lung and Blood Institute. *Clinical Guidelines on the Identification, Evaluation, and Treatment of Overweight and Obesity in Adults: The Evidence Report.* 1998.

CAN A PATIENT OF NORMAL BODY WEIGHT, A NORMAL SERUM CHOLESTEROL LEVEL, AND NO HISTORY OF DIABETES HAVE FATTY LIVER DISEASE?

Arun J. Sanyal, MD

Metabolic syndrome as defined by dyslipidemia, diabetes mellitus, and obesity is almost universally associated with nonalcoholic fatty liver disease (NAFLD). The driving force behind the phenotypic expression of both metabolic syndrome and NAFLD is insulin resistance (IR). While typically IR is associated with diabetes, obesity, and dyslipidemia, it may be present in individuals with no overt expression of metabolic syndrome. It has also been seen that patients with familial insulin resistance syndrome who are often nonobese and have high prevalence of not only NAFLD but also known to progress nonalcoholic steatohepatitis (NASH) and cirrhosis.

Retrospective and autopsy studies have shown that NAFLD and NASH are more common in obese individuals than in lean individuals.[1] It is also well known that diabetes mellitus and dyslipidemia are present in up to one third of patients who have been diagnosed with NASH.[2,3] However, it has also been shown that IR state can be independent of one or more components of metabolic syndrome phenotype and may manifest primarily with hepatic steatosis.

The process of developing the IR state is complex and is dependent on a complex array of events, including genetic predisposition, lifestyle issues, and interplay of proinflammatory and anti-inflammatory cytokines and hormones. In the Asian population, although the incidence of glucose intolerance and fatty liver disease is high, the rate of obesity is low. Similarly, although obesity, dyslipidemia, and glucose intolerance is common in the African American population, the incidence of NAFLD is low. Numerous studies have demonstrated the importance of central or visceral adiposity rather than generalized obesity to the process of IR. Hence, although obesity is a common phenotypic presentation of metabolic syndrome, it is not necessary for IR state to manifest.

Insulin Resistance States in Nonobese

Insulin resistance states unrelated to obesity are seen in congenital and acquired lipodystrophy states. Lipodystrophy states, whether congenital or acquired, are associated with loss of adipose tissues in the arm, legs, and face, with redistribution in truncal areas in some individuals. All of them invariably have IR state, with hepatic steatosis developing eventually. While the mechanism of IR differs between the congenital and the acquired variety, the eventual outcome in terms of development of metabolic syndrome is the same.

Acquired lipodystrophy is seen most commonly in human immunodeficiency virus (HIV)-infected patients who are being treated with protease inhibitors as apart of their antiretroviral therapy. It is estimated that approximately 40% of HIV-infected patients who are receiving protease inhibitors for greater than 1 year develop lipodystrophy.[4,5] These patients usually have redistribution of body fat with loss of adipose tissues in the extremities and deposition in the truncal region. Metabolically, there is a moderate to severe IR state with dyslipidemia but infrequent glucose intolerance. Hepatic steatosis also has been reported to develop in these cohorts of patients.

Non–protease inhibitor–induced acquired lipodystrophy is extremely rare and can either be partial or generalized. Insulin resistance is commonly seen in the generalized form that eventually leads to cirrhosis due to either hepatic steatosis or autoimmune hepatitis. These patients usually have loss of adipose tissues in the extremities and face with occasional redistribution to the truncal aspects.

Congenital lipodystrophy is another extremely rare condition that usually presents at birth with complete loss of adipose tissue and severe insulin resistance. These patients eventually develop hepatic steatosis and cirrhosis.

Finally, and most importantly, a substantial proportion of the general population with a BMI <25 who are not diabetic have biochemical evidence of insulin resistance when tested with a euglycemic hyperinsulinemic clamp. One way to identify such subjects is with a fasting insulin level; typically such individuals have an insulin level in the fourth quartile for their age, gender, and race.

Hence, in summary, IR state leading to hepatic steatosis in absence of the typical obese diabetic phenotype can develop in selected group of individuals with abnormalities in distribution and formation of adipose tissues. While these disorders are rare overall, causes of fatty liver disease, the increased use of antiretroviral agents in HIV-infected patients may make it an important problem.

NAFLD in Nonobese and Nondiabetic

It is well established that the prevalence of NAFLD is higher among overweight people. However, it has also been observed that although the mean body mass index of Asians is lower than that of a matched Western cohort, the prevalence of NAFLD and metabolic syndrome is similar.[6] It is estimated that the prevalence of NAFLD ranges from 13% to 23% in non-obese, non-diabetic individuals, a number that is similar to that seen in the obese diabetic population. The similar prevalence of NAFLD in these two very different phonotypical cohorts may be the result of genetic factors, lifestyle issues, and diet. In addition, it has also been proposed that markers such as waist-hip ratio and waist circumference may be more related to NAFLD than the conventional marker of obesity; ie, body mass index (BMI). Hence, the so-called non-obese populace may have one or more of these abnormal truncal obesity parameters and consequently develop NAFLD in the presence of normal BMI and weight.

It is well known that visceral adipose tissue is more closely linked with insulin resistance metabolic syndrome and hepatic steatosis than peripheral adipose tissue. This is most likely the result of being able to generate greater hepatic free fatty acid load secondary to increased lipolysis. This increased availability of substrate for lipogenesis in the presence of insulin resistance eventually overwhelms the hepatic lipid regulatory pathways and leads to net hepatic lipid deposition. Asians have a higher proportion of visceral fat and a lower lean body mass than comparable Caucasian subjects with the same BMI.[7] It has also been observed that the prevalence of NAFLD is similar in Asians as in Caucasians. Hence, a combination of higher visceral fat and high carbohydrate diet in the presence of genetic predisposition toward metabolic syndrome may lead to hepatic steatosis despite normal body weight.

In summary, it can be stated that IR is the sine qua non of NAFLD and is commonly associated with the obese phenotype. However, this is not universal and individuals with normal body weight may have IR and consequently develop NAFLD. As pathogenesis of IR is multifactorial, it may be that one or more factors, such as genetics and distribution of body fat, besides lifestyle may set one up to develop NAFLD.

References

1. Wanless IR, Lentz JS. Fatty liver hepatitis (steatohepatitis) and obesity: an autopsy study with analysis of risk factors. *Hepatology.* 1990;12:1106-1110.
2. James OF, Day CP. Non-alcoholic steatohepatitis (NASH): a disease of emerging identity and importance. *J Hepatol.* 1998;29:495-501.
3. Cortez-Pinto H, Camilo ME, Baptista A, De Oliveira AG, De Moura MC. Non-alcoholic fatty liver: another feature of the metabolic syndrome? *Clin Nutr.* 1999;18:353-358.
4. Ene L, Goetghebuer T, Hainaut M, Peltier A, Toppet V, Levy J. Prevalence of lipodystrophy in HIV-infected children: a cross-sectional study. *Eur J Pediatr.* 2007;166:13-21.
5. Martinez E, Gatell JM. Metabolic abnormalities and body fat redistribution in HIV-1 infected patients: the lipodystrophy syndrome. *Curr Opin Infect Dis.* 1999;12:13-19.
6. Das UN. Metabolic syndrome X is common in South Asians, but why and how? *Nutrition.* 2002;18:774-776.
7. Dudeja V, Misra A, Pandey RM, Devina G, Kumar G, Vikram NK. BMI does not accurately predict overweight in Asian Indians in northern India. *Br J Nutr.* 2001;86:105-112.

SECTION VI

CHOLESTATIC LIVER DISEASE

WHEN SHOULD I INITIATE TREATMENT WITH URSODEOXYCHOLIC ACID AND WHAT DOSE SHOULD I UTILIZE IN MY PATIENT WITH PRIMARY BILIARY CIRRHOSIS?

Puneet Puri, MD
Velimir A. Luketic, MD

Primary biliary cirrhosis (PBC) is a chronic cholestatic liver disease that primarily affects middle-aged women. The progressive injury in PBC is a 2-step process that begins with immune-mediated destruction of the microscopic intrahepatic bile ducts and subsequent retention of bile constituents, including bile salts, within the liver. Bile salts are powerful detergents that damage cells both by directly disrupting cell and organelle membranes and by activating intracellular signals promoting apoptosis. In PBC, the result of cholangiocyte and hepatocyte injury is self-perpetuating liver damage that leads to progressive fibrosis and, eventually, cirrhosis and ultimately end-stage liver disease. The rate at which this process occurs and the disease progresses varies from patient to patient and depends on complex interaction of as yet poorly understood patient and environmental factors. As a result, the initial presentation of PBC can rage widely: in 2007, more than half of patients are asymptomatic at the time of diagnosis; when symptoms are present, fatigue and pruritus are the most common; rarely, ascites, hepatic encephalopathy, or esophageal variceal hemorrhage are the first manifestation of PBC.

The asymptomatic or early phase of PBC is associated with detection of antimitochondrial antibody (AMA) and cholestatic pattern of liver enzyme abnormalities. The duration of asymptomatic phase is extremely variable and can be as long as 20 years; the mean, however, is about 6 years, and once symptoms develop survival is significantly lower than in a paired control population. This phase correlates with stages I and II found on liver biopsy. In stage I the inflammation is confined to the portal space and is focused on the bile duct; in stage II injury extends into the hepatic parenchyma ("cholate" injury or biliary piecemeal) and is associated with portal fibrous expansion and proliferation of bile ductules. The symptomatic phase is marked by fatigue and pruritus and rarely by jaundice and other symptoms. During the later course of the symptomatic phase, patients may present with signs and symptoms due to portal hypertension. The duration of the symptomatic phase can be as long as 10 years. The mean 5-year survival rate among symptomatic patients is 50% (range 30% to 70%). This phase correlates to histologic stages II and III and, rarely, stage IV. The presence of bridging fibrosis and cirrhosis characterize stages III and IV, respectively. Serum bilirubin levels >2 mg/dL in symptomatic individuals heralds the arrival of the terminal phase and complications of end-stage liver disease. The mean survival of patients in this phase is <3 years unless orthotopic liver transplantation (OLT) is performed. This phase is associated with histological stage IV.

Ursodeoxycholic acid (UDCA) is currently the only approved medical treatment aimed at modifying the natural history of PBC. UDCA is a naturally occurring bile acid that is common in bears—hence *urso*—but found only in low concentrations in humans. Because of the orientation of its hydroxyl groups, UDCA is more hydrophilic and thus a less effective (and less toxic) detergent than its epimer chenodeoxycholate and the other bile acids found in human bile. The mechanisms of action proposed to explain the protective effect of UDCA in PBC include stimulation of biliary secretion, decrease in the cytotoxicity of the overall bile acid pool, and direct protection of membranes from toxic effects of retained hydrophobic bile acids. The latter was thought to be due to the direct interaction between UDCA and cell membranes.[1] More recent data, however, suggest that more important may be UDCA stimulation, via epidermal growth factor receptor, of intracellular survival signaling and thus inhibition of the caspase cascade resulting in decrease in bile acid induced apoptosis.

UDCA also increases the expression and apical insertion of transporter proteins. The consequence is an increase in both export of bile acids from hepatocytes to bile and an increase in bile volume and bile flow. As a result, there is an overall increase in the clearance of potentially toxic bile acids from the liver and thus a decrease in cellular and organelle injury. As a bile acid, UDCA also participates in the enterohepatic circulation of bile salts. When UDCA is given on a regular basis, its percentage of the total bile acid pool expands in a dose-dependent manner and can be as high as 69% (daily dose of 25 to 35 mg/kg).[1] The effect of UDCA administration, therefore, is a bile acid pool that is overall more hydrophilic and thus less toxic to the liver. Several studies have looked at the optimal dose of UDCA for use in PBC: in general, biliary enrichment with UDCA and its effect on biochemical liver tests was the least at doses ≤10 mg/kg/d and became attenuated at doses ≥20 mg/kg/d.[1] The recommended dose of UDCA for use in PBC is 13 to 15 mg/kg/d.

To date, some 20 therapeutic trials involving almost 2000 subjects have evaluated the use of UDCA in PBC. In general, these trials showed that when compared to placebo or no treatment, UDCA improved cholestatic indices (alkaline phosphatase, gamma glutamyl transpeptidase, and bilirubin) and transaminases, less frequently cholesterol and albumin, and almost never symptoms (very rarely pruritus). In one study, UDCA also reduced the rate at which esophageal varices developed, but not the rate of bleeding from varices. When it comes to hard end points—the improvement in histology and survival—the beneficial effect of UDCA has been more difficult to prove and the results mixed.

This is because essentially all the published trials were designed to measure changes in surrogate markers of cholestasis, such as alkaline phosphatase or bilirubin, and as a result are underpowered to measure UDCA impact on survival. When meta-analyses were performed to improve the power to detect small changes not seen in individual studies, the results were also disappointing.[2] Two meta-analyses, one of 8 and the other of 16 randomized controlled trials that included 1114 and 1422 subjects, respectively, concluded that death, liver transplantation (LT), and death or LT were not significantly affected by UDCA. The third meta-analysis excluded trials that used UDCA ≤10 mg/kg/d or lasted ≤2 years. While there was marginally significant reduction in time to death or LT (OR 0.76, $p = 0.05$), most of the benefit came from LT, a relatively soft end point rather than death.

To get around the problem of lack of power, the investigators of the 3 largest trials that had used the same formulation and dose of UDCA, ie, 13 to 15 mg/kg/d, combined the raw data from their 548 patients. The re-analysis was able to show a significant increase in transplant-free survival among those patients who remained on continuous UDCA therapy for 4 years compared to those who initially received placebo and then UDCA.[3] On the basis of this trial, the FDA approved UDCA for treatment of PBC. While the use of LT rather than death as the main end point remains an issue, these are the best data that we are ever likely to get regarding the effect of UDCA therapy on patient survival. As a result, the recommended regimen for PBC is UDCA 13 to 15 mg/kg/d in divided doses.

According to the guidelines published by the American Association for the Study of Liver Disease, all PBC patients with abnormal liver biochemistry should be considered for specific therapy with UDCA.[4] In theory, treatment initiated early in the course of PBC would be of most benefit since, if successful, it would prevent development of potentially irreversible changes such as bridging fibrosis and cirrhosis. To prove this, however, would require a placebo-controlled UDCA trial with either a long follow-up (beginning during stage I or II and continuing into stage IV) or short follow-up with a large number of patients, both of which are currently unattainable. Data from currently available studies, unfortunately, are not helpful: while a study that used UDCA 10 to 12 mg/kg/d suggested that UDCA was less effective in patients whose bilirubin was greater than 2 mg/dL at baseline,[5] the combined data analysis showed the greatest benefit in those with cirrhosis and bilirubin >1.4 mg/dL (albeit more evaluable events were observed in patients with severe rather than with mild disease).[3]

Instead, mathematical modeling has been used to predict disease outcome and/or pre-transplantation survival with fair degree of accuracy. A recently published study[6] examined the effect of UDCA therapy on the natural history of PBC using a multistate continuous-time Markov model with following study end points: (a) histologic progression, (b) OLT, and (c) death. A cohort of 262 PBC patients was treated with UDCA (13 to 15 mg/kg per day) and prospectively followed for a mean duration of 8 years (range 1 to 22). The survival rate of UDCA-treated PBC patients with early disease (stage I/II) was comparable to age-matched and sex-matched controls (RR = 0.8, $p = 0.5$). Those with advanced disease (stage III/IV), on the other hand, had shorter survival without OLT compared to the controls (RR = 2.2, $p < 0.05$) despite UDCA therapy. This study added 2 important pieces of information: it described the natural course of PBC in the UDCA era, and it showed that UDCA normalized the patient survival rates when given at an early histologic stage. Therefore, it is recommended that UDCA therapy be initiated early during the course of PBC.

What follows are some general principles that may be helpful in the management of patients on UDCA. UDCA is a well-tolerated drug. The most common side effect is diarrhea, which often resolves with more frequent administration of smaller doses. Compliance with a single UDCA dose each day, however, is likely to be better, and in PBC the biliary enrichment with once a day dosing is similar to that seen in divided doses. In some patients, UDCA therapy has been associated with weight gain that occurs in the first 12 months of treatment, persists for the duration of treatment, and is independent of baseline BMI. This should be discussed with patients before initiating UDCA therapy. Many PBC patients suffer from pruritus and are prescribed cholestyramine. Cholestyramine can also bind other medications, including UDCA, and patients should be warned to take cholestyramine 3 to 4 h before or after any other drug. Finally, if liver function tests do not improve significantly after 6 months of UDCA therapy, the patient should be reevaluated for compliance or presence of an overlap syndrome (autoimmune hepatitis) or an unrelated cholestatic disorder.

In summary, we recommend that all PBC patients should be treated with UDC at the dose of 13 to 15 mg/kg/d. The therapy should be initiated at diagnosis and continued indefinitely. While UDCA slows the progression of PBC and improves survival in treated patients, its use does not lead to resolution of the disease. Those who progress to end-stage liver disease in spite of UDCA therapy should be evaluated for transplantation.

References

1. Paumgartner G, Beuers U. Mechanisms of action and therapeutic efficacy of ursodeoxycholic acid in cholestatic liver disease. *Clin Liver Dis.* 2004;8:67-81.
2. Shi J, Wu C, Lin Y, Chen Y-X, Zhu L, Xie W. Long-term effects of mid-dose ursodeoxycholic acid in primary biliary cirrhosis: a meta-analysis of randomized controlled trials. *Am J Gastroenterol.* 2006;101:1529-1538.
3. Poupon, RE, Lindor, KD, Cauch-Dudek, K, Dickson ER, Poupon R, Heathcote EJ. Combined analysis of randomized controlled trials of ursodeoxycholic acid in primary biliary cirrhosis. *Gastroenterology.* 1997;113:884-890.
4. Heathcote EJ. Management of primary biliary cirrhosis. The American Association for the Study of Liver Diseases practice guidelines. *Hepatology.* 2000;31:1005-1013.
5. Combes B, Carithers RL, Maddrey WC, et al. A randomized, double-blind, placebo-controlled trial of ursodeoxycholic acid in primary biliary cirrhosis. *Hepatology.* 1995;22:759-766.
6. Corpechot C, Carrat F, Bahr A, Chretien Y, Poupon RE, Poupon R. The effect of ursodeoxycholic acid therapy on the natural course of primary biliary cirrhosis. *Gastroenterology.* 2005;128:297-303.

WHAT TYPE OF TESTING DOES MY PATIENT WITH PRIMARY BILIARY CIRRHOSIS REQUIRE?

Velimir A. Luketic, MD

Primary biliary cirrhosis (PBC) is a chronic cholestatic liver disease characterized by immune-mediated destruction of the small, intrahepatic (intralobular and septal) bile ducts. Loss of bile ducts results in accumulation of bile constituents within the liver that cause hepatocyte injury, fibrosis, and cirrhosis and, ultimately, end-stage liver disease.[1] When PBC was first described in the 1850s, cirrhosis was usually already present and the typical patient was a middle-aged woman with itching. Today most patients are asymptomatic at presentation and are identified when an elevated alkaline phosphatase, found during routine testing.[2] The diagnosis of PBC therefore depends on confirmation that cholestasis is present, exclusion of other cholestatic disorders, the presence of anti-mitochondrial antibodies (AMA), and the typical histologic findings.

Confirming the Presence of Cholestasis

Evaluation of cholestasis begins with the detection of an elevated serum alkaline phosphatase (ALP) level.[2] In the liver, ALP is primarily a canalicular enzyme and is present in the bile at high concentrations. In cholestasis, ALP appearance in the blood is due the disruption of intercellular tight junctions between hepatocytes and/or cholangiocytes permitting (a) regurgitation of bile contents from the biliary tree to the sinusoids via a paracellular pathway and (b) migration of canalicular enzymes from the basolateral membrane to the entire hepatocyte membrane. In patients with PBC, ALP is usually at least 1.5 times the upper limit of normal; it can, however, be within normal limits in early PBC and particularly in AMA-positive asymptomatic relatives of PBC patients. The clinical setting is usually sufficient to confirm that ALP is of liver origin. If there is doubt—bone, intestine, and placenta are other common sources—ALP isoenzymes or 5'-nucleotidase, another canalicular enzyme, can be checked.[2] The most practical method to confirm liver as the source of the abnormal ALP level is to test for gamma-glutamytransferase (GGT), an enzyme that in serum is almost entirely of hepatobiliary origin.

Other Laboratory Studies

In patients with PBC I also routinely check transaminases, bilirubin, albumin, and pro-thrombin time (PT). Aspartate (AST) and alanine (ALT) aminotransferase are intracellular enzymes that "leak" across a damaged cell membrane; abnormal serum levels therefore are considered markers of hepatocyte injury. In PBC, AST and ALT are either normal or mildly elevated. Significant elevations—more than 5 times upper limit of normal—raise the possibility that the patient has a primary hepatocellular disorder, eg, acute viral hepatitis, or that the primary biliary cirrhosis/autoimmune hepatitis (PBC/AIH) overlap is present. In either case, additional testing including a liver biopsy is required.

Elevated serum bilirubin is a marker of advanced PBC. Bilirubin values greater than 2.5 mg/dL are indicative of poor prognosis and serum bilirubin and albumin levels and PT are integral components of Mayo Natural History Model for PBC (which can be found at http://www.mayoclinic.org/gi-rst/models.html). In addition, an elevated prothrombin time that corrects with vitamin K is strongly suggestive of fat malabsorption due to lack of bile acids in patients with cholestasis. This maneuver obviates the need to test for low vitamin K levels in those with advanced PBC. Such patients should, however, have vita-min D levels tested (preferably 25-hydroxyvitamin D) to help with the management of osteoporosis commonly seen in women who have PBC (bone densitometry should also be performed). Vitamins E and A are rarely deficient in PBC and testing serum levels is not required.

In common with other cholestatic liver diseases, PBC patients tend to have elevated cholesterol values. The cause is regurgitation of lipid-rich vesicles across the disrupted canalicular and cholangiolar tight junctions. Labeled *lipoprotein X*, these vesicles migrate with low-density lipoprotein (LDL) fraction and contribute to an abnormal lipid profile that may be the first indication that cholestasis is present. Routine testing for markers of hemochromatosis, Wilson's disease, and alpha-1-antitrypsin deficiency is not indicated in suspected PBC since these disorders rarely present as cholestasis. An abnormal angio-tensin-converting enzyme (ACE) level, however, could initiate a search for sarcoidosis isolated to the liver and an elevated alpha-fetoprotein may direct further search for an infiltrating hepatocellular carcinoma (absent other evidence for its presence) or metastatic cancer. Nonalcoholic steatohepatitis can present as an isolated elevation of alkaline phos-phatase and an abnormal glycohemoglobin may be the only indicator of its presence.

Serologies

Presence of a high AMA titer in a woman with cholestasis is virtually diagnostic of PBC. AMA is usually identified by indirect tissue immunoflorescence using rat stomach or kidney.[3] The method is simple and cheap but can result in false-positive readings due to errors in localization. In addition, what is considered a high titer will vary from lab to lab. The targets of AMA have been identified as lipoyl domains of the 2-oxoacid dehydrogenase complex located on the inner mitochondrial membrane that includes pyruvate, 2-oxoglutarate, and branched-chain 2-oxoacid dehydrogenases. Enzyme-linked immunosorbent assay (ELISA) and immunoblot assays using these antigens have shown AMA to have a specificity and sensitivity for PBC that are greater than 95% and may be even greater if all the immunoglobulin fractions are examined. AMA may be present in significant titers even before development of symptoms and laboratory abnormalities; histology in such patients is frequently abnormal and symptomatic disease develops in all.

As many as 70% of PBC patients also have elevated serum IgM, a finding that can be helpful in making the diagnosis in difficult cases. At least another 50% of PBC patients are also anti-nuclear (ANA) and anti–smooth muscle (ASMA) antibody positive.[1] In most instances, ANA and ASMA titers are low; in the setting of a positive AMA on the other hand, high titres of either ANA and/or ASMA, an elevated IgG, and moderately abnormal transaminases raise the possibility that the patient has a PBC/AIH overlap syndrome. A biopsy is required to make the diagnosis. Finally, 5% to 10% of patients have so-called AMA-negative PBC: clinical, biochemical, and histologic findings are consistent with PBC, but AMA is negative and ANA, ASMA, and IgG titers are high. The diagnosis is made by biopsy and confirmed by positive response to ursodiol.[2]

In an acute setting, intrahepatic cholestasis may be a sign of a viral illness. Most common are infectious mononucleosis and cytomegalovirus (CMV), and in questionable cases appropriate testing should be performed. In addition, one should never forget that both hepatitis A and, to a lesser extent, hepatitis B can follow a primarily cholestatic, sometimes relapsing course characterized by severe pruritus. All patients with PBC should be tested for exposure to hepatitis A and hepatitis B, not the least to see whether vaccination is needed.

Radiologic Assessment of Bile Ducts

Every patient with biochemical tests suggestive of cholestasis should have a radiologic examination.[4] Ultrasound (US) is particularly good at differentiating between intrahepatic (eg, PBC) and extrahepatic biliary tract disease (dilated ducts secondary to obstruction) and gall bladder pathology. It is also very good at detecting focal lesions within the liver—lesions as small as 1 cm can be identified in spite of extensive parenchymal disease due to fat or cirrhosis—and it can accurately differentiate between cystic (cysts, abscesses, septated cystadenomas) and solid lesions (tumors). US is therefore the preferred modality when screening cirrhotics, including PBC patients, for hepatocellular carcinoma. Because of imaging characteristics, US is not effective at differentiating among solid hepatic lesions such as hepatoma, adenoma, or focal nodular hyperplasia; computed tomography (CT) or magnetic resonance imaging (MRI) is required for that. Direct cholangiographic (endoscopic or magnetic resonance) imaging of the bile ducts is rarely required in PBC and is reserved for the situations where the diagnosis is uncertain; eg, a male with typical clinical, biochemical, and histologic findings of PBC but a negative AMA requires a cholangiogram to rule out the diagnosis of primary sclerosing cholangitis.

Liver Biopsy

Historically, the definitive diagnosis of PBC required the presence of AMA in the serum, ALP elevation for at least 6 months, and liver biopsy findings compatible with the disease. A probable diagnosis of PBC could be made if 2 of the 3 criteria were met. A recent retrospective analysis of a large sample of patients, however, showed that a combination of a positive AMA, ALP level > 1.5 times upper limit of normal, and AST < 5 times upper limit of normal had a positive predictive value of 98.2% for the diagnosis of PBC.[5] Argument has therefore been made that liver biopsy should be reserved for those who do not meet the above criteria.

I feel that a biopsy at the time of diagnosis continues to be of value. It provides a baseline against which response to treatment can be evaluated. Further, staging, ie, determining the extent of fibrosis, has prognostic value in PBC beyond that available from indices based on noninvasive testing. Thus, identification of bridging fibrosis or cirrhosis in a patient without clinical evidence of portal hypertension can help identify need for additional diagnostic measures such as US screening for hepatocellular carcinoma and endoscopic screening for varices. Biopsy findings may also be the only way to differentiate PBC from infiltrating disorders such as lymphoma, sarcoidosis (also characterized by granulomatous destruction of bile ducts), metastatic or primary hepatocellular carcinoma, and amyloidosis; nonalcoholic fatty liver disease; small duct primary sclerosing cholangitis; and idiopathic adulthood ductopenia. It is also required to make the diagnosis of suspected PBC/AIH overlap, AMA negative cholestasis, and suspected viral infection.

Summary

I would recommend the following tests in patients with PBC:
1. Initial visit:
    a.   ALP, AST, ALT, bilirubin, albumin, PT/INR, CBC with platelets
    b.   AMA, ANA, ASMA, anti-HAV total, anti-HBV core IgG, anti-HBV surface
    c.   ultrasound
    d.   liver biopsy (elective but recommended)
2. Follow-up:
    a.   ALP, AST, ALT, bilirubin, albumin, PT/INR, CBC with platelets, AFP (if indicated)
    b.   serum vitamin D, bone densitometry (if indicated)
    c.   upper endoscopy to screen for varices (if indicated)
    d.   ultrasound to screen for hepatocellular carcinoma (if indicated)
3. Diagnosis in doubt (choice of test will depend on clinical setting):
    a.   liver biopsy (required)
    b.   IgM, IgG, HCV, CMV serologies, EBV serologies
    c.   CT, MRI, MRCP, ERCP

References

1. Kaplan MM, Gershwin ME. Primary biliary cirrhosis. *N Engl J Med*. 2005;353:1261-1273.
2. Leuschner U. Primary biliary cirrhosis—presentation and diagnosis. *Clin Liver Dis*. 2003;7:741-758.
3. Bogdanos DP, Baum H, Vergani D. Antimitochondrial and other autoantibodies. *Clin Liver Dis*. 2003;7:759-777.
4. Heathcote EJ. Management of primary biliary cirrhosis. *Hepatology*. 2000;31:1005-1013.
5. Zein CO, Angulo P, Lindor KD. When is liver biopsy needed in the diagnosis of primary biliary cirrhosis? *Clin Gastroenterol* Hepatol. 2003;1:89-95.

Is Ursodeoxycholic Acid Effective for the Treatment of Primary Sclerosing Cholangitis?

B. Marie Reid, MD
Velimir A. Luketic, MD

Primary sclerosing cholangitis (PSC) is a progressive cholestatic liver disease characterized by inflammation and obliterative fibrosis of the intrahepatic and extrahepatic biliary tree. The causes for the initial bile duct injury remain largely unknown. Proposed mechanisms include genetic predisposition, immunologic abnormalities, bacterial proteins from the enterohepatic circulation, chronic viral infections, and ischemia. Progressive disease, however, is thought to be due to the development of cholestasis and retention of hydrophobic bile salts within the liver. Bile salt–mediated injury to cholangiocytes and hepatocytes in turn results in the development of fibrosis, cirrhosis, and, ultimately, end-stage liver disease. The course of PSC in any one individual is unpredictable—bacterial infections and development of a dominant stricture can accelerate disease progression—but worldwide the median survival of patients with PSC has been documented to be 10 to 12 years.[1]

There is no commonly accepted medical treatment for PSC. The interest in ursodeoxycholic acid (UDCA) as therapy of PSC stems from its successful use in other cholestatic diseases, specifically primary biliary cirrhosis (PBC). The rationale for UDCA use in PSC is the same as in PBC (see Question 31 for discussion). Both PBC and PSC are cholestatic disorders in which hydrophobic bile acids retained within the liver are responsible for progressive disease. As a hydrophilic bile acid, UDCA is the least effective detergent and therefore the least toxic constituent of the bile acid pool. When given in pharmacologic doses, UDCA becomes proportionately the most common bile acid in the enterohepatic circulation, thus decreasing the overall toxicity of the bile acid pool. By stimulating bile flow it also increases the clearance of toxic hydrophobic bile acids from the liver. Finally, UDCA has been shown to modulate both the proapoptotic and antiapoptotic intracellular pathways, thus decreasing the bile acid–induced hepatocyte and cholangiocyte injury.

The first study to evaluate the effectiveness of UDCA in PSC was an open label trial in which 12 subjects received UDCA 10 mg/kg/d for 30 months.[1] Published in 1991, it reported improvements in both liver enzymes and symptoms (histology was not evaluated) and encouraged initiation of larger randomized controlled trials. The results from 6 such trials (total of 261 subjects) using varying amounts of UDCA (10 mg/kg/d, 13 to 15 mg/kg/d, and fixed doses of 600 and 750 mg/d) were published during the 1990s. Although these trials confirmed the beneficial effect of UDCA on biochemical liver tests, none showed improvements in symptoms or (more importantly) histology.[2] Further, even the largest trial (105 subjects randomized) was insufficiently powered to adequately measure UDCA effect on survival. The same disappointing results were obtained by a meta-analysis of 5 of the studies (183 subjects): when compared to placebo or no treatment, UDCA significantly improved biochemical liver tests including bilirubin and transaminases, but not albumin; however, UDCA however was not shown to significantly reduce the risk of death, frequency of treatment failure (liver transplantation, varices, ascites, encephalopathy), liver histologic deterioration, or cholangiographic deterioration.[3]

The meta-analysis as well as some of the individual studies was criticized because a significant proportion of the subjects received UDCA at doses ≤10 mg/kg/d. As indicated previously (see Question 31 for discussion) the optimal dose of UDCA in PBC is thought to be 13 to 15 mg/kg/d. Experience in other cholestatic diseases, eg, cystic fibrosis associated cholestasis, suggests that even higher doses may be required for UDCA to be effective.[1] The rationale for use of higher doses of UDCA is based on an observation that with worsening cholestasis the UDCA enrichment of the bile acid pool declined and that higher doses of UDCA were required to achieve the same level of enrichment.[4] A recent study of the biliary bile acid composition of 56 patients with PSC, however, showed that biliary enrichment with UDCA increases with increasing dose but that the effect may plateau at 22 to 25 mg/kg/d with enrichment of 58.6%.[1] Thus, the optimal dose of UDCA in PSC has yet to be determined.

Three studies have explored the use of UDCA at doses as high as 30 mg/kg/d. In a pilot study, 30 subjects with PSC were treated with UDCA 25 to 30 mg/kg/d for 1 year. Liver biochemistries improved significantly and when these were used to determine the subject prognosis (the Mayo Natural History Model for PSC can be found at http://www.mayoclinic.org/gi-rst/models.html), the expected mortality at 4 years would have declined from 17% to 11%.[1] The second trial randomized 26 subjects to UDCA 20 mg/kg/d or placebo. After 2 years there was significant improvement in liver biochemistries, cholangiographic appearance of the biliary tree, and liver fibrosis as assessed by disease staging.[4] The largest recent trial compared UDCA 17 to 23 mg/kg/d and placebo in 219 subjects for up to 5 years. While there were fewer deaths, liver transplantations, and cholangiocarcinomas in the UDCA-treated group, the differences when compared to placebo were not statistically significant.[5] Thus, in spite of the relatively large number of subjects recruited, the study remained underpowered. The trend toward survival benefit in the UDCA-treated group, however, is encouraging, especially if, as seems likely from previous discussion, the dose of UDCA was too low to adequately enrich the bile acid pool. Currently, a National Institutes of Health–sponsored, multicenter placebo-controlled trial of UDCA 25 to 30 mg/kg/d is underway and by 2010 should answer the question of whether UDCA should be used in PSC.

In summary, UDCA has been shown to improve biochemical abnormalities in patients with PSC. Since this effect is irrespective of the dose, I usually start all my patients with PSC on 13 to 15 mg/kg/d (the dose most frequently used in controlled trials). To date, however, there is no evidence that UDCA, whatever the dose, improves survival or delays time to liver transplantation. While higher doses of UDCA ultimately may be shown to improve histology and cholangiographic appearance of bile ducts (20 mg/kg/d), improve prognosis as calculated by Mayo PSC model (25 to 30 g/kg/d), or decrease the frequency of death, transplantation, and cholangiocarcinoma (17 to 23 mg/kg/d), the study proving that has not yet been completed. Thus, at this time I cannot recommend the routine use of high-dose UDCA in patients with PSC.

References

1. Sandhu BS, Luketic VA. Management of primary sclerosing cholangitis. *Gastroneterol Hepatol.* 2006;2:843-849.
2. Cullen SN, Chapman RW. The medical management of primary sclerosing cholangitis. *Semin Liver Dis.* 2006;26:52-61.
3. Chen W, Gluud C. Bile acids for primary sclerosing cholangitis (review). *Cochrane Database Syst Rev.* 2004;3: CD004036.
4. Mitchell SA, Bansi DS, Hunt N, et al. A preliminary trial of high-dose ursodeoxycholic acid in primary sclerosing cholangitis. *Gastroenterology.* 2001;121:900-907.
5. Olsson R, Boberg KM, de Muckadell OS, et al. High-dose ursodeoxycholic acid in primary sclerosing cholangitis: a 5-year multicenter, randomized, controlled study. *Gastroenterology.* 2005;129:1464-1472.

SHOULD I BE SCREENING MY PATIENTS WITH PRIMARY SCLEROSING CHOLANGITIS FOR CHOLANGIOCARCINOMA?

Michael Fuchs, MD, PhD, FEBG

The natural history of primary sclerosing cholangitis (PSC) is typically one of progressive cholestasis eventually leading to jaundice and end-stage liver disease. The overall median survival of patients is in the range of 10 to 12 years. Since current drug therapy is unsatisfactory, with scant evidence of benefit, liver transplantation is the treatment of choice for end-stage disease, with excellent outcomes improving long-term survival.[1]

PSC is now considered as a premalignant disease, with the majority of patients developing cholangiocellular, colon, or pancreatic cancer. Up to 36% of patients develop cholangiocarcinoma (CCA) with an estimated annual incidence of 1% and a 20% lifetime risk.[2] Recent studies showed that smoking, alcohol, older age at onset of PSC, chronic bile duct infections, and longer history of ulcerative colitis before diagnosis of PSC may increase the risk of developing CCA.[3] However, the majority of carcinomas arise in the absence of any of these risk factors.

Early stage CCA can be treated successfully with liver transplantation resulting in excellent outcomes. Because the majority of patients with PSC will not develop CCA, liver transplantation, with its mortality and morbidity, is not justified in a preemptive manner. Therefore, early and reliable detection of malignancy is warranted. An ideal CCA screening test in the setting of available effective early treatment that improves outcome should (a) have a high sensitivity and specificity, (b) be simple and safe to perform, (c) be broadly available at a reasonable cost, and (4) be acceptable to the patient and physician.

Unfortunately the diagnosis of CCA remains a challenging task, especially when multiple diagnostic tests performed yield conflicting results. The mainstays of diagnosing CCA are noninvasive imaging studies such as magnetic resonance (MR) cholangiography, computed tomography, and positron emission tomography. Endoscopic retrograde cholangiography and endoscopic ultrasonography offer the possibility to obtain tissue for histology and cytology to confirm diagnosis, whereas laparoscopy is used for staging only. Unfortunately, currently available serological tests such as CA 19-9 can only reliably confirm advanced CCA but are useless for screening purposes.[4]

A combination of dynamic contrast-enhanced magnet resonance imaging and MR cholangiography does provide not only information about the liver parenchyma but also detects bile duct changes. Thus, this modality is ideal for visualization of intrahepatic and extrahepatic CCA, which appear as hypointense lesions on T1-weighted images and hyperintense lesions on T2-weighted images. Images can be enhanced employing super-paramagnetic iron and delayed gadolinium images.[5] New multislice three-dimensional spiral computed tomography cholangiography (3-D CTC) may be useful in patients with mildly elevated bilirubin (<2 mg/dL) for whom MR cholangiography is contraindicated. CT angiography is also superb for detecting vascular encasement.[6] Whether dynamic positron emission tomography with ^{18}F-fluoro-2-deoxy-D-glucose[7] may be utilized to detect early CCA has to be studied in more detail. However, one has to keep in mind that a normal positron emission tomography does not allow exclusion of cancer for certain, especially in the case of a CCA of the ductal infiltrative type.

The pathogenesis of CCA likely involves a multiple-step progression from normal biliary epithelium to dysplastic and malignant change, dyplasia being the main precursor of an invasive carcinoma. Thus, endoscopic retrograde cholangiography with the possibility of tissue sampling (eg, biopsy, brush cytology) appears to be the most promising technique to identify PSC patients with CCA precursor lesions, which should have a great impact on survival.[8] However, the inflammatory nature of PSC presents inherent difficulties in specimen procurement and cytologic interpretation, resulting in a low sensitivity of standard brush cytology. Reasons for wide differences in sensitivity in brush cytology include variations in factors like sampling, quality of the cytological material, interpretation, and the expertise of the pathologist. Also, it has been shown that CCA may develop outside dominant strictures from which normally tissue will be sampled. It may be possible to enhance the sensitivity cytology by combining biliary brush cytology with fluorescence in situ hybridization[9] and digital image analysis techniques,[10] thereby avoiding false-positive results. The value of optical coherence tomography for identifying dysplastic or early malignant changes of the biliary tract in patients with PSC has to be determined.[11]

Endoscopic ultrasound allows visualization of the biliary tree and guided lymph node fine needle aspiration facilitates assessment of resectability or eligibility for transplantation. One has to bear in mind that periportal lymphadenopathy is a common finding in patients with PSC and does not represent an indicator of malignancy.

In summary, there is scant evidence that currently used tests to approach surveillance for CCA are effective in prolonging patient survival. Therefore, routine screening of patients with PSC cannot be advocated outside of prospective clinical trials at this time.

References

1. Levy C, Lindor KD. Primary sclerosing cholangitis: epidemiology, natural history, and prognosis. *Semin Liver Dis.* 2006;1:22-30.
2. Burak K, Angulo P, Pasha TM, Egan K, Petz J, Lindor KD. Incidence and risk factors for cholangiocarcinoma in primary sclerosing cholangitis. *Am J Gastroenterol.* 2004;99:523-526.

3. Malhi H, Gores GJ. Review article: the modern diagnosis and therapy of cholangiocarcinoma. *Aliment Pharmacol Ther.* 2006;23:1287-1296.
4. Levy C, Lymp J, Angulo P, Gores GJ, LaRusso N, Lindor KD. The value of serum CA 19-9 in predicting cholangiocarcinomas in patients with primary sclerosing cholangitis. *Dig Dis Sci.* 2005;50:1734-1740.
5. Braga HJ, Imam K, Bluemke DA. MR imaging of intrahepatic cholangiocarcinoma: use of ferumoxides for lesion localization and extension. *AJR Am J Roentgenol.* 2001;177:111-114.
6. Zandrino F, Curone P, Benzi L, Ferretti ML, Musante F. MR versus multislice CT cholangiography in evaluating patients with obstruction of the biliary tract. *Abdom Imaging.* 2005;30:77-85.
7. Prytz H, Keiding S, Björnsson E, et al. Dynamic FDG-PET is useful for detection of cholangiocarcinoma in patients with PSC listed for liver transplantation. *Hepatology.* 2006;44:1572-1580.
8. Boberg KM, Jebsen P, Clausen OP, Foss A, Aabakken L, Schrumpf E. Diagnostic benefit of biliary brush cytology in cholangiocarcinoma in primary sclerosing cholangitis. *J Hepatol.* 2006;45:568-574.
9. Kipp BR, Stadheim LM, Halling SA, et al. A comparison of routine cytology and fluorescence in situ hybridizytion for the detection of malignant bile duct strictures. *Am J Gastroenterol.* 2004;99:1675-1681.
10. Baron TH, Harewood GC, Rumalla A, et al. A prospective comparison of digital image analysis and routine cytology for the identification of malignancy in biliary tract strictures. *Clin Gastroenterol Hepatol.* 2004;2:214-219.
11. Singh P, Chak A, Willis JE, Rollins A, Sivak MV. In vivo optical coherence tomography of the pancreatic and biliary ductal system. *Gastrointest Endosc.* 2005;62:970-974.

SHOULD ALL PATIENTS WITH SUSPECTED PRIMARY SCLEROSING CHOLANGITIS UNDERGO AN ENDOSCOPIC RETROGRADE CHOLANGIOGRAPHY TO CONFIRM THIS DIAGNOSIS?

Michael Fuchs, MD, PhD, FEBG

Primary sclerosing cholangitis (PSC) is a rare chronic cholestatic liver disease characterized by inflammation, obliteration, and progressive fibrosis of bile ducts. This results in strictures of the intrahepatic and/or extrahepatic biliary tree, ultimately leading to biliary cirrhosis and end-stage liver disease. The disease usually affects men, presents during the fourth and fifth decade of life, and will develop in up to 8% of patients with ulcerative colitis. Interestingly, up to 80% of patients with ulcerative colitis will develop PSC.[1]

PSC can be suspected based on biochemical abnormalities of elevated serum alkaline phosphatase and gamma-glutamyl transpeptidase (GGT) with usually minor elevations in alanine aminotransferase (ALT) and aspartate aminotransferase (AST). Perinuclear antineutrophil cytoplasmic antibodies (pANCA) are present in up to 80% of patients with PSC, but they are not diagnostic. Unfortunately, currently known polymorphisms of inflammatory bowel disease susceptibility genes do not appear to confer risk for PSC, thus excluding them as a diagnostic test.[2] Because there are no serum markers that allow conclusive diagnosis, the major criterion for diagnosis is the cholangiographic finding of multifocal strictures and beading of the bile ducts. Secondary causes of bile duct strictures such as surgery, infections, ischemia, and trauma must be thoroughly excluded.

For imaging of the biliary tree, invasive and noninvasive procedures are available. For many years, endoscopic retrograde cholangiography (ERC) has been considered a diagnostic gold standard, yielding high-quality images of the intrahepatic and extrahepatic bile ducts in the majority of cases.[3] However, ERC is an invasive procedure, putting patients at risk for pancreatitis and cholangitis, which may be greater in patients with PSC than in those with other diagnoses. Several factors, including low infusion pressure, suboptimal positioning of the catheter, preferential filling of the gallbladder, high-grade stricture of the common bile duct, and experience of the endoscopist, contribute to a lesser degree of ductal visualization of the peripheral bile ducts, which may result in underestimation of the degree of the disease.

In recent years, magnetic resonance (MR) cholangiography techniques[4,5] have improved significantly, offering an alternative to ERC in early diagnosis of PSC. Compared with ERC, this procedure is noninvasive, does not require sedation of the patient, and is without radiation exposure. Another advantage of MR cholangiography is that it allows visualization of peripheral bile ducts in patients with high-grade strictures of the common bile duct or with biliary-enteric anastomosis and gastric bypass procedures. In addition, this imaging technique allows visualization of morphological changes of bile ducts as well as of the hepatic parenchyma associated with PSC. Compared with ERC, nondilated peripheral bile ducts are not well visualized in healthy persons due to the lower spatial resolution of MR cholangiography. However, in the presence of strictures with prestenotic dilatations, these ducts become better visualized, allowing MR cholangiography to be more sensitive than ERC to detect early changes in patients with primary sclerosing cholangitis. Despite the advantages of MR cholangiography, there are some limitations of this procedure. The presence of a bile duct stent or pneumobilia as a result of previous biliary-enteric surgery or ERC can obscure ductal visualization in those ducts. In patients with cirrhosis, regenerative nodules may compress bile ducts, which then are not visualized by MR cholangiography. Finally, the noninvasive nature of the procedure does not allow access for interventional procedures such as biopsies, dilatations of bile duct strictures, and stent placement.

Other imaging studies of the biliary tree such as dynamic ^{99m}Tc hepato-iminodiacetic acid (HIDA) single photon emission tomography,[6] endoscopic ultrasonography,[7] and transpapillary cholangioscopy[8] may be a valuable adjunct to MR cholangiography and ERC but have to be studied in more detail. Of these techniques, endoscopic ultrasonography and cholangioscopy may have the potential to identify early changes of bile duct morphology. In contrast, laparoscopy will only detect advanced stages of the disease, typically presenting with liver surface irregularity, discoloration, and dilation of lymph vessels,[9] and therefore will not play a role in diagnosing PSC.

In summary, MR cholangiography is first choice as a screening test for PSC. However, when there is clinical suspicion that the patient will benefit from therapeutic interventions, ERC is the preferred initial procedure. Under conditions where MR cholangiography is less sensitive and provides equivocal results, ERC is indicated as next diagnostic step (Figure 35-1). It is hoped that advances in proteomics and genomics will ultimately lead to highly sensitive and specific diagnostic tests for diagnosis of PSC.

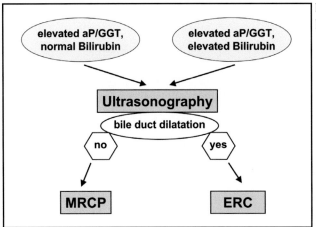

Figure 35-1. Work-up for suspected primary sclerosing cholangitis.

References

1. Levy C, Lindor KD. Primary sclerosing cholangitis: epidemiology, natural history, and prognosis. *Semin Liver Dis.* 2006;1:22-30.
2. Karlsen TH, Hampe J, Wiencke K, et al. Genetic polymorphisms associated with inflammatory bowel disease do not confer risk for primary sclerosing cholangitis. *Am J Gastroenterol.* 2007;102:115-121.
3. Moff SL, Kamel IR, Eustace J, et al. Diagnosis of primary sclerosing cholangitis: a blinded comparative study using magnetic resonance cholangiography and endocopic retrograde cholangiography. *Gastrointest Endosc.* 2006;64:219-223.
4. Fulcher AS, Turner MA, Franklin KJ, et al. Primary sclerosing cholangitis: evaluation with MR cholangiography—a case-control study.
5. Vitellas KM, Enns, RA, Keogan MT, et al. Comparison of MR cholangiopancreaticographic techniques with contrast-enhanced cholangiography in the evaluation of sclerosing cholangitis. *AJR Am J Roentgenol.* 2002;178:327-334.
6. Jonas E, Hultcrantz R, Slezak P, Blomqvist L, Schnell PO, Jacobsson H. Dynamic 99m Tc-HIDA SPET: noninvasive measuring of intrahepatic bile flow: description of the method and a study in primary sclerosing cholangitis. *Nucl Med Commun.* 2001;22:127-134.
7. Mesenas S, Vu C, Doig L, Meenan J. Duodenal EUS to identify thickening of the extrahepatic biliary tree wall in primary sclerosing cholangitis. *Gastrointest Endosc.* 2006;63:403-408.
8. Tischendorf JJ, Kruger M, Trautwein C, et al. Cholangioscopic characterization of dominant bile duct stenoses in patients with primary sclerosing cholangitis. *Endoscopy.* 2006;38:665-669.
9. Ikeda F, Yamamoto K, Fujioka S, et al. Laparoscopic findings in primary sclerosing cholangitis. *Endoscopy.* 2001;33:267-270.

36

MY PATIENT WITH ULCERATIVE COLITIS RECENTLY UNDERWENT A TOTAL COLECTOMY FOR SEVERE DYSPLASIA. DOES THIS REDUCE THE RISK THAT HE WILL GET PRIMARY SCLEROSING CHOLANGITIS?

Michael Fuchs, MD, PhD, FEBG

Forty-two years ago, the association between primary sclerosing cholangitis (PSC) and ulcerative colitis (UC) was described and confirmed by investigators around the world. UC can be diagnosed at any time during the course of PSC, and vice versa. In general, UC is diagnosed several years earlier than PSC and PSC may even develop following colectomy for UC.[1] Epidemiological studies demonstrated that the prevalence of UC in patients with PSC varies from 21% to 80%.[2] This strongly supports screening colonoscopy for patients with PSC. The prevalence of PSC in patients with UC, however, is much lower and varies from 0.5% to 7.5%.[2] The presence of enlarged perihepatic lymph nodes by abdominal ultrasonography and colitis beyond the left side of the colon should prompt screening for PSC, especially if elevations for alkaline phosphatase are documented.

While PSC in patients without UC is not a separate entity from PSC in patients with UC, UC in patients with PSC appears to have a more quiescent course.[3] Also, rectal sparing and backwash ileitis are more common in UC patients with PSC. In addition, UC patients with PSC are more likely to develop pouchitis following ileal pouch–anal anastomosis and this is not improved by liver transplantation.

UC is a well-established risk factor for developing colorectal cancer. Recently, it has become evident that PSC increases the risk of colorectal cancer in UC patients, especially when the disease duration is beyond 10 years.[4] It is more difficult to assess whether PSC patients with UC are at higher risk for colorectal cancer than PSC patients without UC. This is due to the fact that assessment of the onset of UC, with its more quiescent course, is difficult. Nevertheless, a recent meta-analysis supports the fact that PSC is an independent risk factor for development of colorectal cancer in patients with UC.[5] PSC patients with UC remain at increased risk for colorectal cancer following liver transplantation,[6] supporting colonoscopic surveillance of transplanted patients. One also has to keep in mind that PSC patients may develop UC for the first time following liver transplantation.[7]

It has not yet been shown convincingly that the current treatment of PSC with ursodeoxycholic acid improves long-term survival. Nevertheless, there is good evidence that ursodeoxycholic acid does reduce the risk of developing colorectal dysplasia.[8]

In summary, the interactions between PSC and ulcerative colitis are complex and incompletely understood. Therefore, it is critical to always consider that a UC patient may develop PSC over time and that liver transplantation does not exclude the patient developing UC with its long-term risks.

References

1. Fausa O, Schrumpf E, Elgjo K. Relationship of inflammatory bowel disease and primary sclerosing cholangitis. *Semin Liver Dis*. 1991;11:31-39.
2. Broome U, Bergquist A. Primary sclerosing cholangitis, inflammatory bowel disease, and colon cancer. *Semin Liver Dis*. 2006;26:31-41.
3. Lundqvist K, Broome U. Differences in colonic disease activity in patients ith ulcerative colitis with and without primary sclerosing cholangitis: a case control study. *Dis Colon Rectum*. 1997;40:451-456.
4. Broome U, Löfberg R, Veress B, Eriksson LS. Primary sclerosing cholangitis and ulcerative colitis: evidence for increased neoplastic potential. *Hepatology*. 1995;22:1404-1408.
5. Soetikno RM, Lin OS, Heidenreich PA, Young HS, Blackstone MO. Increased risk of colorectal neoplasia in patients with primary sclerosing cholangitis and ulcerative colitis: a meta-analysis. *Gastrointest Endosc*. 2002;56:48-54.
6. Vera A, Gunson BK, Ussatoff V, et al. Colorectal cancer in patients with inflammatory bowel disease after liver transplantation for primary sclerosing cholangitis. *Transplantation*. 2003;75:1983-1988.
7. Haagsma EB, van den Berg AP, Kleibeuker JH, Slooff MJ, Dijkstra G. Inflammatory bowel disease after liver transplantation: the effect of different immunosuppressive regimens. *Aliment Pharmacol Ther*. 2003;18:33-44.
8. Pardi DS, Loftus EV, Kremers WK, Keach J, Lindor KD. Ursodeoxycholic acid as a chemopreventive agent in patients with ulcerative colitis and primary sclerosing cholangitis. *Gastroenterology*. 2003;124:889-893.

SECTION VII

CIRRHOSIS

37

WHICH ASYMPTOMATIC PATIENTS WITH CIRRHOSIS SHOULD UNDERGO AN UPPER ENDOSCOPY TO DETERMINE WHETHER THEY HAVE ESOPHAGEAL VARICES?

Nagib Toubia, MD
Adil Habib, MD
Douglas M. Heuman, MD

In our practice, all patients with cirrhosis are offered endoscopy to assess for presence and size of varices. Patients with bridging fibrosis on biopsy may also merit screening endoscopy if they exhibit thrombocytopenia, splenomegaly, or other signs of portal hypertension. We do this for 3 key reasons: (1) esophageal variceal bleeding can occur at any point after development of portal hypertension and carries significant risk; (2) at the present time only endoscopy can reliably detect varices and predict the likelihood of variceal bleeding; and (3) available treatments can prevent variceal bleeding and reduce mortality in high-risk patients.[1]

Preventing variceal hemorrhage is an important goal of management of patients with cirrhosis. Esophageal varices develop in up to two thirds of patients with cirrhosis, and 25% to 40% of all patients with varices will develop variceal hemorrhage. Each episode of active variceal hemorrhage is associated with at least a 20% mortality.[2] Unlike other complications of cirrhosis, variceal bleeding is purely a complication of portal hypertension and can occur without warning in patients with otherwise well-compensated liver function. Also, unlike other complications of cirrhosis, variceal bleeding is abrupt and often catastrophic and can lead to sudden, unexpected out-of-hospital death.

Varices develop when increased pressure and flow in the portal vein cause expansion of collateral channels between the portal and systemic circulation. A critical threshold pressure gradient of about 12 mmHg between these systems is required for varices to form. Intravariceal pressure, increased vessel size and thinning of the vessel wall all contribute to increasing variceal wall tension, according to LaPlace's law:

$$\text{Tension} = \text{Pressure} \times \text{radius/wall thickness}$$

Figure 37-1. Endoscopic view showing large varices of the distal esophagus.

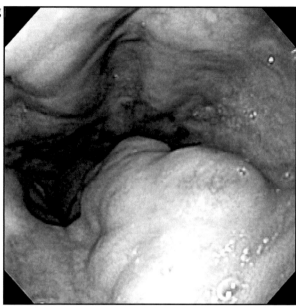

With increasing wall tension, areas of weakness develop in the vessel wall where superficial venules feed into the varix, forming endoscopically visible stigmata (red walls, hematocystic spots). Like blisters on a balloon tire, these areas of weakness can rupture abruptly, producing a "blowout."

Numerous studies show that the risk of bleeding from esophageal varices can be predicted based on their endoscopic appearance. If varices are absent or small and stigmata are absent, risk of variceal hemorrhage is low; with increasing variceal size or stigmata, risk increases progressively.[3] While assessment of variceal size is semiquantitative and somewhat subjective (Figure 37-1), clinical trials indicate that experienced endoscopists in the community setting can reliably distinguish between low-risk and high-risk varices based on their appearance, and this assessment is the single strongest predictor of bleeding risk.[4] Other clinical parameters such as cirrhosis severity (Child-Turcotte-Pugh class), presence of tense ascites, and coagulopathy also affect bleeding risk but to a lesser degree.

In patients with high-risk varices, several treatments have been shown to reduce the risk of variceal hemorrhage and may prolong survival. The best established of these is use of nonselective beta-blockers: propranolol, nadolol, or timolol.[5] These act mainly at the level of the mesenteric arterioles to block vasodilatory beta-1-adrenergic receptors. The resulting increase in mesenteric resistance causes a drop in pressure downstream in the portal vein. The response of portal pressure to beta-blockers is variable and is not clearly related to the systemic effects, so the usual practice is to push the dosage to the limits of tolerance, generally defined as a resting pulse less than 60. Isosorbide mononitrate may provide some synergy with beta-blockers. Band ligation of esophageal varices is also effective and has been advocated as primary prophylaxis by some groups. However, banding in a small percentage of cases may be complicated by massive delayed variceal hemorrhage, and fatalities from this complication have occurred. For this reason, we usually reserve banding for patients at high risk who cannot tolerate effective doses of beta-blockers or patients who have already experienced a variceal bleed, and current guidelines support this approach.[1,6] Transjugular intrahepatic portosystemic shunting (TIPS) is very effective at lowering portal pressure and preventing variceal hemorrhage, but the cost and complication rate are too high to justify its use in primary prophylaxis.

Determination of hepatic venous pressure gradient (a measure of portal pressure in patients with cirrhosis) is favored by some groups as part of routine management of cirrhosis, but it is not universally practiced. The procedure is invasive, requiring jugular puncture with placement of a cannula in the hepatic vein to measure free and wedged pressures. Reliable interpretation of pressure tracings requires some experience and attention to details of technique.[7] A gradient less than 12 mmHg places the patient at low likelihood of variceal bleeding, but higher pressures correlate only weakly with variceal size and bleeding risk. The most important use of this test is to assess response of portal pressure to therapeutic interventions. Patients in whom hepatic venous pressure gradient falls by more than 20% or drops below 12 mmHg with propranolol therapy have excellent results and low risk of bleeding, whereas patients in whom pressure fails to respond remain at risk and may require further prophylaxis with band ligation.[8]

What about follow-up surveillance endoscopy? In asymptomatic cirrhotic patients without varices on initial evaluation, varices subsequently develop at an annual rate of 5% to 15%. Small varices progress to large varices at a rate of 4% to 10% each year. Prophylactic administration of beta-blockers to patients with small varices does not prevent progression to large varices and is associated with significant side effects.[9] Our current practice is to repeat endoscopy at 2-year to 3-year intervals in cirrhotic patients who initially are free of varices, and at 1-year to 2-year intervals in patients with small varices. Large varices are most likely to be found in patients with clinical evidence of portal hypertension, including platelet count less than 100,000/mm^3, elevated INR, or dilated portal vein greater than 13 mm in diameter on ultrasonography.[10] In the absence of these indicators, screening endoscopy may not be cost-effective.[11] The technique of wireless capsule endoscopy has recently been adapted for evaluation of esophageal varices and may eventually replace traditional endoscopy for this indication.[12] Once large varices have been identified and prophylaxis has been initiated, further surveillance is not of proven value.

References

1. Garcia-Tsao G, Wongcharatrawee S. Treatment of patients with portal hypertension and cirrhosis. Literature review and summary of treatment recommendations. Available at: http://www.hepatitis.va.gov/pdf/va01-pr/prtop-08/prtop08-01-gd-01.pdf.
2. D'Amico G, De FR. Upper digestive bleeding in cirrhosis. Post-therapeutic outcome and prognostic indicators. *Hepatology*. 2003;38:599-612.
3. Prediction of the first variceal hemorrhage in patients with cirrhosis of the liver and esophageal varices. A prospective multicenter study. The North Italian Endoscopic Club for the Study and Treatment of Esophageal Varices. *N Engl J Med*. 1988;319:983-989.
4. Merkel C, Zoli M, Siringo S, et al. Prognostic indicators of risk for first variceal bleeding in cirrhosis: a multicenter study in 711 patients to validate and improve the North Italian Endoscopic Club (NIEC) index. *Am J Gastroenterol*. 2000;95:2915-2920.
5. Poynard T, Cales P, Pasta L, et al. Beta-adrenergic-antagonist drugs in the prevention of gastrointestinal bleeding in patients with cirrhosis and esophageal varices. An analysis of data and prognostic factors in 589 patients from four randomized clinical trials. Franco-Italian Multicenter Study Group. *N Engl J Med*. 1991;324:1532-1538.
6. Chalasani N, Boyer TD. Primary prophylaxis against variceal bleeding: beta-blockers, endoscopic ligation, or both? *Am J Gastroenterol*. 2005;100:805-807.

7. Groszmann RJ, Wongcharatrawee S. The hepatic venous pressure gradient: anything worth doing should be done right. *Hepatology.* 2004;39:280-282.

8. D'Amico G, Garcia-Pagan JC, Luca A, Bosch J. Hepatic vein pressure gradient reduction and prevention of variceal bleeding in cirrhosis: a systematic review. *Gastroenterology.* 2006;131:1611-1624.

9. Groszmann RJ, Garcia-Tsao G, Bosch J, et al. Beta-blockers to prevent gastroesophageal varices in patients with cirrhosis. *N Engl J Med.* 2005;24:2254-2261.

10. Schepis F, Camma C, Niceforo D, et al. Which patients with cirrhosis should undergo endoscopic screening for esophageal varices detection? *Hepatology.* 2001;33:333-338.

11. Spiegel BM, Targownik L, Dulai GS, Karsan HA, Gralnek IM. Endoscopic screening for esophageal varices in cirrhosis: is it ever cost effective? *Hepatology.* 2003;37:366-377.

12. Eisen GM, Eliakim R, Zaman A, et al. The accuracy of PillCam ESO capsule endoscopy versus conventional upper endoscopy for the diagnosis of esophageal varices: a prospective three-center pilot study. *Endoscopy.* 2006;38:31-35.

38

I JUST BANDED ACTIVELY BLEEDING VARICES IN A PATIENT WITH KNOWN CIRRHOSIS. THE PATIENT IS NOW HEMODYNAMICALLY STABLE. IS THERE ANYTHING ELSE I SHOULD RECOMMEND?

Nagib Toubia, MD
Adil Habib, MD
Douglas M. Heuman, MD

Variceal bleeding is one of the mosst dramatic and catastrophic problems encountered in the practice of gastroenterology. Achieving initial hemostasis can be a daunting task. The endoscopist has to manage shock and protect the airway while attempting to visualize and ligate pulsing varices immersed in a pool of blood. If you have been able to achieve band ligation and the bleeding has stopped, congratulations—the worst may be over. But you are not quite done yet. Additional short-term measures to consider in this patient are pharmacologic reduction of portal pressure, antibiotic prophylaxis, administration of blood products and clotting factors, and management of concurrent ascites and encephalopathy. You also must be ready to intervene if the patient should rebleed while in the hospital, with measures such as repeat endoscopic band ligation, balloon tamponade, and transjugular intrahepatic portosystemic shunt. Finally, you should establish a plan for long-term management.[1]

Where technically feasible, endoscopic intervention is the preferred approach to achieve immediate control of variceal hemorrhage.[2] Endoscopic hemostatic methods acutely control bleeding by occluding flow in the bleeding varix; if repeated chronically, they prevent variceal rebleeding by producing fibrotic obliteration of the varices that are at greatest risk to rupture. Compared to sclerotherapy, band ligation achieves these goals with less pain and fewer complications (ulceration, esophageal stricture, mediastinitis) and is therefore the preferred approach.[3] Endoscopic injection of cyanoacrylate glue may be preferable for ablation of large gastric varices that are not amenable to banding or sclerotherapy.

Drugs to reduce portal pressure are effective in controlling acute bleeding and reducing the risk of rebleeding.[4] Somatostatin and the somatostatin analogue octreotide reduce portal pressure at least in part by antagonizing the mesenteric vasodilatation that occurs in response to blood in the lumen of the gastrointestinal (GI) tract. Octreotide infusion has few side effects and appears to further reduce the risk of rebleeding when used in conjunction with band ligation.[5] Octreotide also has the advantage of a relatively long half-life; this means that its efficacy is not compromised by transient fluctuations in the rate of infusion, and it can be given by intravenous, intramuscular, or subcutaneous routes. In our patients with variceal bleeding we routinely administer octreotide as a 50-µg intravenous bolus followed by continuous intravenous infusion at 50 µm per hour for 2 to 5 days. Intravenous infusion of arginine vasopressin reduces portal pressure by directly increasing mesenteric arteriolar tone. Because vasopressin also produces systemic vasoconstriction and can precipitate heart failure and myocardial infarction, it should be accompanied by nitroglycerin infusion, which enhances the beneficial effects on portal pressure while reducing cardiovascular complications. This combination has significant side effects and generally should not be continued for more than 24 h.[1] Analogues of vasopressin such as terlipressin have similar efficacy and are safer and easier to use than vasopressin but currently are not available in the United States.

There is considerable controversy regarding criteria for use of blood products and clotting factors in management of cirrhotic bleeding. Overtransfusion during the course of resuscitation may lead to increased portal pressure and increase the risk of recurrent bleeding. Current recommendations call for limiting transfusions of packed red blood cells to the minimum necessary to maintain hematocrit between 25% and 30%.[1] Correction of thrombocytopenia and coagulopathy does not appear to add much to control of variceal hemorrhage beyond the benefits achieved with banding. Platelet transfusions may be given to correct thrombocytopenia, but the benefit is transient at best. We limit platelet transfusion to patients whose platelet counts are less than 75,000/mm[3] and who are at high risk for recurrent bleeding. Excessive transfusion of fresh frozen plasma to correct coagulopathy also can contribute to volume expansion, portal pressure, and risk of rebleeding. Administration of recombinant factor VIIa rapidly corrects coagulopathy without causing volume overload but this treatment is expensive and controlled trials to date have not proven clinical benefit. Vitamin K is routinely given but rarely improves coagulopathy except in cholestatic patients (who may be deficient because they malabsorb fat-soluble vitamins).

Much of the mortality related to variceal hemorrhage comes from infections, including respiratory and urinary infections as well as spontaneous bacterial peritonitis. Aspiration of regurgitated blood leading to aspiration pneumonia can occur even in an alert patient. Furthermore, blood in the gastrointestinal tract leads to a large influx of ammonia and other toxins that aggravate hepatic encephalopathy, producing confusion and somnolence, which increase the risk of aspiration. We usually place a nasotracheal tube before attempting endoscopy or balloon tamponade in the patient with active variceal bleeding. Once the acute bleeding is controlled we administer lactulose via nasogastric tube to help purge residual blood from the gut. This usually leads to improvement in mental status over a period of days. The patient remains intubated until bleeding is controlled and mental status is alert. In addition, all patients with acute variceal hemorrhage should receive prophylactically a broad-spectrum antibiotic such as ceftriaxone or ciprofloxacin. This measure has been shown to reduce secondary infections and mortality.[6] In patients with tense ascites, large volume paracentesis may be worthwhile. Some studies show that this reduces portal pressure, and it clearly improves comfort, respiratory function, nutrition, and mobility, all of which are important for preventing respiratory infections.

With the measures shown above, acute control of variceal bleeding can be achieved in about 85% of cases, with continued satisfactory control at 5 days in over 80%.[7] Treatment failure is more likely if the initial hemorrhage is severe, as judged by indicators such as hypotension, azotemia, or substantial transfusion requirements. Endoscopic features predictive of early recurrence include active bleeding at the time of the initial endoscopy, stigmata of recent bleeding, and large varices. Severity of portal hypertension, measured by the hepatic venous pressure gradient (HVPG), correlates with the risk of recurrent bleeding as well as with survival after an initial variceal hemorrhage, but currently there is no practical way to routinely determine HVPG in the setting of acute hemorrhage.

If the patient should rebleed in the hospital, repeat endoscopic therapy may be successful in many cases. If it fails, the patient may require urgent transjugular intrahepatic portosystemic shunt (TIPS) placement. A portosystemic shunt that reduces the portal-systemic pressure gradient to less than 12 mmHg is highly effective in preventing rebleeding both acutely and chronically, but shunts do not always achieve this goal because of technical problems in stent placement, high portal flow, or subsequent shunt stenosis. TIPS carries substantial procedural risk in the unstable patient, and it increases the frequency and severity of hepatic encephalopathy.[8] Over months to years TIPS may become stenotic and require revision, though the frequency of TIPS stenosis during the first year after placement has decreased from about 50% to less than 20% with the advent of coated stents.

In the patient who rebleeds, balloon tamponade may be useful as a bridge measure to control massive hemorrhage and stabilize patients for repeat endoscopy or TIPS. Balloon tamponade, employing Linton or Blakemore-Sengstaaken tubes, reduces pressure in esophageal varices by compressing the bleeding varix itself or occluding the feeding vessels as they cross the esophagogastric junction. While often temporarily effective, this treatment carries high risk of fatal complications, including aspiration pneumonia and esophageal rupture.[9] Balloon tamponade should not be maintained for more than 48 h because of the risk of epithelial necrosis.

Long-term measures to prevent recurrence of variceal bleeding are referred to as *secondary prophylaxis* (as opposed to primary prophylaxis: preventing the initial variceal bleed). The backbone of secondary prophylaxis is variceal ablation using repeated endoscopic band ligation. Endoscopic treatments must be repeated, typically at intervals of 3 to 6 weeks, until varices are completely thrombosed; thereafter, repeat endoscopy at 6- to 12-month intervals usually is sufficient to identify and treat newly formed varices. Endoscopic treatment reduces the long-term risk of recurrent variceal bleeding by about two thirds. Nonselective beta-blockers (propranolol, nadolol, timolol) are nearly as effective as variceal ligation for chronic prevention of recurrent variceal bleeding (they are not used in the acute setting for fear of blocking compensatory responses to hypovolemic shock). A few studies suggest that combining beta-blockers with serial band ligation further improves control of bleeding,[10,11] though each is so effective alone that it is hard to show added benefit from the combination. Even so, we know that beta-blockers work, and they are inexpensive and relatively safe. We routinely give a beta-blocker to patients who have bled from varices until variceal obliteration is complete, and if the drug is well tolerated, we continue it indefinitely.

The ultimate intervention for control of variceal hemorrhage is liver transplantation, which normalizes portal pressure and hepatic function. However, transplantation today is rarely necessary to achieve control of variceal bleeding. Among patients referred for consideration of liver transplantation, a history of prior variceal hemorrhage does not increase the risk of pretransplant death. Except in rare circumstances, variceal bleeding does not justify exceptional priority for transplantation.

References

1. Garcia-Tsao G, Wongcharatrawee S. Treatment of patients with portal hypertension and cirrhosis. Literature review and summary of treatment recommendations. Available at: http://www.hepatitis.va.gov/pdf/va01-pr/prtop-08/prtop08-01-gd-01.pdf.
2. Grace ND. Diagnosis and treatment of gastrointestinal bleeding secondary to portal hypertension. American College of Gastroenterology Practice Parameters Committee. *Am J Gastroenterol.* 1997;92:1081-1091.
3. Laine L, Cook D. Endoscopic ligation compared with sclerotherapy for treatment of esophageal variceal bleeding. A meta-analysis. *Ann Intern Med.* 1995;123:280-287.
4. Banares R, Albillos A, Rincon D, et al. Endoscopic treatment versus endoscopic plus pharmacologic treatment for acute variceal bleeding: a meta-analysis. *Hepatology.* 2002;35:609-615.
5. Corley DA, Cello JP, Adkisson W, Ko WF, Kerlikowske K. Octreotide for acute esophageal variceal bleeding: a meta-analysis. *Gastroenterology.* 2001;120:946-954.
6. Bernard B, Grange JD, Khac EN, Amiot X, Opolon P, Poynard T. Antibiotic prophylaxis for the prevention of bacterial infections in cirrhotic patients with gastrointestinal bleeding: a meta-analysis. *Hepatology.* 1999;29:1655-1661.
7. D'Amico G, De FR. Upper digestive bleeding in cirrhosis. Post-therapeutic outcome and prognostic indicators. *Hepatology.* 2003;38:599-612.
8. Boyer TD. Transjugular intrahepatic portosystemic shunt: current status. *Gastroenterology.* 2003;124:1700-1710.
9. Avgerinos A, Klonis C, Rekoumis G, Gouma P, Papadimitriou N, Raptis S. A prospective randomized trial comparing somatostatin, balloon tamponade and the combination of both methods in the management of acute variceal haemorrhage. *J Hepatol.* 1991;13:78-83.
10. Lo GH, Lai KH, Cheng JS, et al. Endoscopic variceal ligation plus nadolol and sucralfate compared with ligation alone for the prevention of variceal rebleeding: a prospective, randomized trial. *Hepatology.* 2000;32:461-465.
11. de la PJ, Brullet E, Sanchez-Hernandez E, et al. Variceal ligation plus nadolol compared with ligation for prophylaxis of variceal rebleeding: a multicenter trial. *Hepatology.* 2005;41:572-578.

WHICH PATIENTS WITH CHRONIC LIVER DISEASE SHOULD I SCREEN FOR HEPATOCELLULAR CARCINOMA?

Douglas M. Heuman, MD
Adil Habib, MD

In our practice we recommend that patients with established cirrhosis of any cause undergo screening for hepatocellular carcinoma (HCC)*. We also screen patients who have lesser degrees of liver fibrosis on biopsy if there is evidence of portal hypertension (for example, thrombocytopenia or splenomegaly) or compromised liver function (abnormal albumin, INR, or bilirubin), since biopsy can sometimes underestimate severity of liver disease. Finally, we screen for hepatocellular carcinoma in adult patients with long-standing chronic hepatitis B infection regardless of the severity of liver fibrosis.

We follow this algorithm with the full understanding that benefits of screening have not been proven unequivocally by controlled clinical trials,[1] its cost-effectiveness in different populations is unknown, and a significant minority of gastroenterologists and hepatologists are unconvinced of its benefits.[2] Nonetheless, screening is so widely practiced that it has become the de facto standard of care and has been incorporated into consensus guidelines.[3]

The rationale for screening rests on 3 considerations. First, a population at high risk of hepatocellular carcinoma can be identified. Second, noninvasive tests exist that can detect hepatocellular cancer at early stages. And third, cases diagnosed early can be cured in many cases by liver transplantation, surgical resection, or locoregional therapy such as radiofrequency ablation, while cases diagnosed at later stages usually cannot be treated definitively and have poor outcomes.

A prerequisite for screening is identification of a population at risk. In the case of hepatocellular carcinoma, the major predisposing condition is hepatic cirrhosis. As in other conditions associated with chronic injury and repair, the progression to cancer in

---

*Technically only the initial testing constitutes screening, while subsequent periodic repeat testing is termed surveillance, but for the sake of simplicity we will use the term *screening* here to include both.

cirrhosis reflects repeated cell division in response to inflammatory injury and selection of mutant clones resistant to apoptosis. In patients with cirrhosis caused by chronic hepatitis C, risk of cirrhosis is on the order of 1.5% to 5% per year. Similar risk is seen in patients with chronic hepatitis B, hemochromatosis, alcoholic cirrhosis, and nonalcoholic steatohepatitis.[4] The risk of HCC in cirrhosis caused by other conditions such as alpha-1-antitrypsin deficiency, autoimmune hepatitis, and primary biliary cirrhosis is less well defined but clearly exists. Although cancer incidence probably is higher in patients with more advanced cirrhosis, all cirrhotics are at risk, and most liver cancers occur in patients with compensated cirrhosis. Even when cirrhosis is so subtle as to be unrecognized clinically, patients are at risk for cancer.

In hepatitis B, the risk of cancer is only partly related to cirrhosis; many cases occur in patients without significant fibrosis. It is thought that integration of hepatitis B virus (HBV) DNA into the host genome at random sites may lead to activation of oncogenes and disruption of key tumor-suppressor genes. Risk of cancer is related to disease activity and the level of hepatitis B viremia, and there is preliminary data to suggest that antiviral therapy with interferon or nucleosides may reduce the cancer risk. At the present time we continue to screen all patients with chronic hepatitis B surface antigenemia, but a good case can be made for limiting screening to patients with significant fibrosis and/or high viral load, especially in areas where hepatitis B is endemic and health care resources are limited.

Other factors also affect cancer risk. Within all groups, cancer incidence increases with age and duration of disease. Risk also is several-fold greater in males than females. For this reason, in some guidelines, screening is recommended only for males greater than age 40 or females greater than age 50. However, we prefer at this point not to exclude younger adult patients from screening, since their potential for curative treatment and years of life to be gained through early intervention are greater than with older patients. Family history of hepatocellular carcinoma is another strong risk factor and may be a consideration in screening decisions, especially among younger or non-cirrhotic patients.

Having identified a patient at risk, what are the tools available to us for early detection of hepatocellular carcinoma? These fall into two categories: imaging and laboratory markers. Most studies of hepatocellular carcinoma surveillance have employed ultrasound imaging. Ultrasound is widely available, inexpensive, and noninvasive. In the non-cirrhotic patient, it is very sensitive for detecting cancer nodules as small as one centimeter. Standard practice currently calls for ultrasound at 6-month to 12-month intervals for HCC surveillance.[3] Unfortunately, ultrasound is operator dependent, and in the setting of cirrhosis ultrasound has difficulty separating incipient cancers from cirrhotic nodules. More sophisticated tests such as computed tomography or magnetic resonance imaging, especially when combined with multiphase contrast imaging, are more accurate, but they are also more costly. As a compromise we routinely perform surveillance imaging at 6-month intervals, alternating ultrasound with 3-phase contrast computed tomography.

A number of tumor markers detectable in the circulation may provide clues to the presence of hepatocellular carcinoma. Alpha fetoprotein (AFP), the best known, is a protein normally synthesized by the embryonic liver and also commonly produced by hepatocellular carcinomas. Circulating levels of AFP are abnormally elevated (greater than 20 ng/mL) at the time of HCC diagnosis in about 2 out of 3 of cases. However, AFP must be interpreted with caution. AFP elevations also are seen in the absence of cancer in 15% to 20% of patients with active cirrhosis. Even very high levels of AFP are not completely specific; among 22 patients with negative imaging and AFP > 500 who were transplanted for presumed hepatocellular carcinoma, only 6 were found to have cancer in the explanted liver.[5] In addition, AFP elevations tend to be associated with more aggressive tumors that have poorer prognosis, so even if screening with AFP leads to earlier detection of some cancers, it may not improve overall outcomes very much. Despite these limitations, we routinely check AFP at 3-month to 6-month intervals in patients we are screening for HCC, and when AFP levels rise we obtain additional imaging tests. Two new HCC markers have recently become available in the United States: AFP-L3% and DCP (des-gamma carboxy prothrombin). The role of these newer markers in surveillance is not yet clear.[6]

Screening clearly allows diagnosis of hepatocellular carcinoma at earlier stages. This is important because prognosis for long-term disease-free survival following diagnosis of HCC depends upon curative treatment, and likelihood of curative treatment is much better with early stage disease. Small solitary tumors (less than 2 cm in diameter) often can be eradicated by locoregional therapy such as radiofrequency ablation, but as lesions become larger, the likelihood of cure with this modality diminishes. For solitary lesions confined to a single lobe, radical surgical resection (typically hepatic lobectomy) can be curative, and this is the treatment of choice in many patients with good liver function. In native Alaskans with chronic hepatitis B followed since the 1970s with period determination of AFP, 23 of 32 patients whose HCC was identified through AFP elevation were able to undergo resection and 42% were alive at 5 years, compared to no 5-year survival among unscreened historical controls.[7] A large prospective randomized controlled trial in China[8] found that, compared to unscreened patients, individuals screening with AFP and ultrasound at 6-month intervals were much more likely to have HCC diagnosed at an early stage and were 6 times more likely to undergo resection for HCC; 5-year survival of cancer patients in the screened group was 46% versus 0% in the unscreened group.

Cirrhotic patients with portal hypertension and/or compromised hepatic function have limited hepatic reserve and their outcomes after hepatectomy are poor. For these patients, total hepatectomy and liver transplantation is often the best option. Mazzaferro and colleagues from Milan were the first to demonstrate that transplantation provides excellent results for cirrhotic patients with hepatocellular carcinoma when restricted to patients with early stage disease. Since 1996 in the United States, patients meeting the so-called Milan criteria have received expedited priority for liver transplantation. However, livers for transplantation are a scarce resource. Because likelihood of post-transplant cancer recurrence and death increases at more advanced tumor stage, current regulations in the United States preclude liver transplantation in most patients whose liver cancers have progressed beyond the Milan criteria. Thus, diagnosis of hepatocellular carcinoma at an early stage is a critical determinant of access to transplantation.

Even when hepatocellular carcinoma is found at an early stage, curative treatment cannot always be offered. Transplantation or surgical resection may carry prohibitive risk in many patients with severe heart or lung disease, extrahepatic malignancy, or very advanced age. Even more limited locoregional ablation often is precluded in patients with advanced cirrhosis or severe comorbid disease. In such individuals, screening is unlikely to be of benefit and may reasonably be withheld.

References

1. Sherman M, Peltekian KM, Lee C. Screening for hepatocellular carcinoma in chronic carriers of hepatitis B virus: incidence and prevalence of hepatocellular carcinoma in a North American urban population. *Hepatology.* 1995;22:432-438.
2. Chalasani N, Said A, Ness R, Hoen H, Lumeng L. Screening for hepatocellular carcinoma in patients with cirrhosis in the United States: results of a national survey. *Am J Gastroenterol.* 1999;94:2224-2229.
3. Bruix J, Sherman M. Management of hepatocellular carcinoma. *Hepatology.* 2005;42:1208-1236.
4. el-Serag HB. Epidemiology of hepatocellular carcinoma. *Clin Liver Dis.* 2001;5:vi, 87-107.
5. Kemmer N, Neff G, Kaiser T, et al. An analysis of the UNOS liver transplant registry: high serum alpha-fetoprotein does not justify an increase in MELD points for suspected hepatocellular carcinoma. *Liver Transpl.* 2006;12:1519-1522.
6. Spangenberg HC, Thimme R, Blum HE. Serum markers of hepatocellular carcinoma. *Semin Liver Dis.* 2006;26:385-390.
7. McMahon BJ, Bulkow L, Harpster A, et al. Screening for hepatocellular carcinoma in Alaska natives infected with chronic hepatitis B: a 16-year population-based study. *Hepatology.* 2000;32(pt 1):842-846.
8. Zhang BH, Yang BH, Tang ZY. Randomized controlled trial of screening for hepatocellular carcinoma. *J Cancer Res Clin Oncol.* 2004;130:417-422.

SHOULD I VACCINATE MY PATIENTS WITH CIRRHOSIS FOR HEPATITIS A AND B?

Douglas M. Heuman, MD
Adil Habib, MD

This is an easy one. All patients with liver disease should be offered immunization against viral hepatitis A and B, unless they are already known to be immune. Why? Because it works; because it is inexpensive; because the consequences of acute viral hepatitis in a patient with chronic liver disease could be devastating; because it is standard of care; and because, like your grandmother's chicken soup, "It couldn't hurt."

It appears that acute viral hepatitis in patients with preexisting liver disease carries a higher than usual risk of liver failure and death. The evidence for this, summarized recently by Keeffe,[1] is largely based on retrospective epidemiological studies. For example, following hepatitis A outbreaks in Shanghai and the United States during the 1980s, patients with chronic hepatitis B had a 5-fold to 30-fold increased risk of death compared to patients without liver disease. Vento and colleagues[2] presented a retrospective series of 17 patients with chronic hepatitis C who developed acute hepatitis A; 7 developed fulminant hepatic failure and 6 died. The latter risks may have been overstated, as larger prospective population studies do not confirm this high risk of liver failure in hepatitis C patients exposed to hepatitis A. Less literature is available regarding acute hepatitis B superinfection in patients with chronic liver disease, but what there is suggests a more severe course.[3] National consensus panels in the United States have recommended routine immunization for both hepatitis A and B in patients with hepatitis C and other chronic liver diseases.[4,5]

Effective vaccines for hepatitis B have been available for over 25 years in the United States and hepatitis A vaccines for 10 years. A combined vaccine covering both viruses (Twinrix) also is available. The available preparations and recommended schedules are shown in Table 40-1. The earliest hepatitis B vaccines were prepared using hepatitis B surface antigen isolated from human blood, but all current hepatitis vaccines employ viral

Table 40-1

Hepatitis A and B Vaccines: Available Preparations and Recommended Schedules for Adult Patients With Normal Immune Function*

Virus	Vaccine	Dosage	Schedule
HAV	HAVRIX (SmithKline Beecham)	1440 units in 1 mL	2 doses: 0 and 6 to 12 months
HAV	VAQTA (Merck)	50 units in 1 mL	2 doses: 0 and 6 months
HBV	Energix-B (SmithKline Beecham)	20 mcg in 1 mL	3 doses: 0, 1 to 2, and 4 to 6 months
HBV	Recombivax HB (Merck)	10 mcg in 1 mL	3 doses: 0, 1 to 2, and 4 to 6 months
Both	Twinrix	720 units (A) and 20 mcg (B) in 1 mL	3 doses: 0, 1, and 6 to 12 months

*Adapted from http://digestive.niddk.nih.gov/ddiseases/pubs/vaccinationshepab/

proteins produced by recombinant or cell culture technology.[6] The vaccines are given by simple intramuscular (IM) injection. The timing for follow-up injections is not critical and can be lengthened to suit the convenience of physician and patient. Charges average about $60 per injection ($80 for Twinrix). Patients with mild chronic liver disease respond normally to hepatitis A and B vaccines, but patients with decompensated liver cirrhosis are less likely to respond.[7]

When we first see a patient with liver disease, we routinely check the status of immunity to hepatitis A and B. Immunity to hepatitis A is indicated by a positive serum test for total antibody to hepatitis A virus, while immunity to hepatitis B is indicated by total antibody to hepatitis B surface antigen. Be careful what you order: many of the serology panels employed to evaluate the patient with suspected acute hepatitis measure only IgM antibodies, not total (IgG plus IgM). After vaccination we recheck these markers to confirm that immunity has been achieved. In vaccine nonresponders who are at significant risk, especially cirrhotics, it may be reasonable to repeat a course of immunization, perhaps employing higher or more frequent doses as recommended for patients with immune-deficiency states.[8] Patients who do not respond to immunization should be counseled to avoid behaviors and situations that might expose them to infection with hepatitis A or B.

References

1. Keeffe EB. Acute hepatitis A and B in patients with chronic liver disease: prevention through vaccination. *Am J Med.* 2005;118(suppl 10A):21S-27S.

2. Vento S, Garofano T, Renzini C, et al. Fulminant hepatitis associated with hepatitis A virus superinfection in patients with chronic hepatitis C. *N Engl J Med.* 1998;338:286-290.

3. Liaw YF, Yeh CT, Tsai SL. Impact of acute hepatitis B virus superinfection on chronic hepatitis C virus infection. *Am J Gastroenterol.* 2000;95:2978-2980.

4. National Institutes of Health Consensus Development Conference Panel statement: management of hepatitis C. *Hepatology.* 1997;26(suppl 1):2S-10S.

5. Fiore AE, Wasley A, Bell BP. Prevention of hepatitis A through active or passive immunization: recommendations of the Advisory Committee on Immunization Practices (ACIP). *MMWR Recomm Rep.* May 2006;55:1-23.

6. Davis JP. Experience with hepatitis A and B vaccines. *Am J Med.* 2005;118(suppl 10A):7S-15S.

7. Lau DT, Hewlett AT. Screening for hepatitis A and B antibodies in patients with chronic liver disease. *Am J Med.* 2005;118(suppl 10A):28S-33S.

8. Laurence JC. Hepatitis A and B immunizations of individuals infected with human immunodeficiency virus. *Am J Med.* 2005;118(suppl 10A):75S-83S.

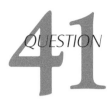

A HEALTHY PATIENT NOT KNOWN TO HAVE CHRONIC LIVER DISEASE, WITH NORMAL LIVER CHEMISTRIES AND LIVER FUNCTION, WAS FOUND TO HAVE A 4-CENTIMETER LIVER MASS ON ULTRASOUND. SHOULD I BIOPSY THIS?

Douglas M. Heuman, MD
Adil Habib, MD

The answer to this simple question is unfortunately rather complicated. Biopsy plays an important role in diagnostic evaluation of liver masses, but it is not always necessary and may be harmful. The decision to biopsy, like all other decisions in medicine, requires balancing of risks and benefits.[1] Compared to routine percutaneous liver biopsies performed for evaluation of liver disease, biopsies of liver masses carry a higher risk of hemorrhage. This is especially true for highly vascular tumors. Spread of malignant cells along the needle track is well documented with biopsy of hepatocellular carcinoma, though the risk of this is less than 10% and probably closer to 1%. Most important, a negative biopsy does not exclude the possibility of cancer, and failure to appreciate this fact may lead to fatal delay in treatment.

Given these risks, it is desirable to try to establish a diagnosis of a liver mass by noninvasive means where possible, especially if the lesion is likely to be benign. Where potentially curable hepatic malignancy is strongly suspected, it sometimes may be better to proceed directly to resection or liver transplantation. This is not to say that percutaneous biopsy must be avoided: it is often critically important for arriving at a diagnosis.[2] But the decision of who, what, and when to biopsy requires some clinical judgment.

Liver masses fall into three general categories: benign lesions, metastases of extrahepatic malignancies, and primary hepatic malignancies and their precursors (dysplastic nodules). Noninvasive clinical evaluation can often allow one to distinguish reliably among these possibilities.

The most common benign hepatic tumor is a cavernous hemangioma. These almost always are asymptomatic and can be managed expectantly; biopsy carries high risk of bleeding and should be avoided. Cavernous hemangioma usually can be diagnosed on imaging studies. Small lesions have a typical ultrasound appearance. Larger lesions exhibit a characteristic pattern of vascular perfusion, with nodular contrast enhancement beginning peripherally and progressing centrally and with slow washout of contrast. While nuclear medicine blood pool scans have traditionally been employed to make this distinction, similar information can be gained from multiphase contrast computed tomography (CT) and magnetic resonance imaging (MRI) or by angiography. Other benign hepatic tumors such as focal nodular hyperplasia also have typical radiographic appearance. Some benign lesions may be hard to distinguish radiographically from malignancy; when unsure, biopsy may be required.[3]

Metastases to the liver from extrahepatic malignancies are very common. Most are multiple, but they can be solitary. Tumors that frequently metastasize to the liver include lung, breast, colon, pancreas, stomach, and melanoma. In most cases, a careful history and physical exam will provide hints of the possible primary, including risk factors such as smoking, symptoms, and physical findings. A CT scan of the chest and abdomen usually will provide additional clues (for example, a thickening of the wall of the stomach or colon, a lung or pancreatic mass, mesenteric lymphadenopathy, or adrenal metastases). If liver metastasis is suspected, biopsy of the hepatic mass is sometimes the most efficient way to establish a diagnosis of cancer and can provide clues to the primary site. However, it may be preferable in many cases to pursue the primary lesion instead, especially if bronchogenic, colonic, or gastric cancer is suspected.

Primary hepatic malignancies and their precursors, dysplastic nodules, occur mostly in the setting of cirrhosis, though noncirrhotic patients with chronic hepatitis B also are at risk. In a patient with an unexpected finding of a liver mass on imaging, we would look closely for subtle signs of cirrhosis. These may include laboratory studies (low platelets, elevated ratio of aspartate transaminase to alanine transaminase) or findings on diagnostic imaging (increased parenchymal echogenicity, prominent left and caudate hepatic lobes, splenomegaly).[4] We also would evaluate for common causes of liver disease such as past alcoholism, nonalcoholic steatohepatitis, hepatitis B, hepatitis C, and hemochromatosis. Finally we would determine serum level of alpha fetoprotein. If all of these are negative, then primary hepatocellular cancer is less likely.

Primary hepatocellular carcinomas are usually vascular tumors and derive their blood supply entirely from the hepatic artery, rather than the portal vein. This gives them a characteristic radiographic appearance on dynamic imaging studies such as 3-phase contrast CT or MRI. In the arterial phase, the lesion enhances relative to the surrounding liver; in the portal venous phase, the lesion becomes hypodense. When this pattern of enhancement is seen in a lesion exceeding 2 cm in diameter, in a patient with cirrhosis, and especially if it is accompanied by markedly elevated alpha fetoprotein, hepatocellular carcinoma can be diagnosed with high reliability and biopsy may be unnecessary.[5,6] About 20% of hepatocellular carcinomas have atypical imaging features, however, and in about one third the alpha fetoprotein is normal. In these cases, diagnosis is less certain and biopsy should be considered.

Since a negative biopsy does not completely rule out the possibility of cancer, some experts would recommend complete excision of any liver lesion that might be a curable cancer (primary or metastatic). If this approach is to be taken, then needle biopsy is unnecessary, since the pathologist will receive the entire lesion for histological examination. For smaller lesions, radiofrequency ablation may be as effective as resection, with less morbidity.[7] Biopsy can be performed in conjunction with radiofrequency ablation; this approach permits cautery of the needle track to reduce the risk of bleeding or tumor seeding.

References

1. Campbell MS, Reddy KR. Review article: the evolving role of liver biopsy. *Aliment Pharmacol Ther.* 2004;20:249-259.
2. Bialecki ES, Ezenekwe AM, Brunt EM, et al. Comparison of liver biopsy and noninvasive methods for diagnosis of hepatocellular carcinoma. *Clin Gastroenterol Hepatol.* 2006;4:361-368.
3. Mortele KJ, Ros PR. Benign liver neoplasms. *Clin Liver Dis.* 2002;6:119-145.
4. Kelleher TB, Afdhal N. Noninvasive assessment of liver fibrosis. *Clin Liver Dis.* 2005;9:vii, 667-683.
5. Bruix J, Sherman M, Llovet JM, et al. Clinical management of hepatocellular carcinoma. Conclusions of the Barcelona-2000 EASL conference. European Association for the Study of the Liver. *J Hepatol.* 2001;35:421-430.
6. Talwalkar JA, Gores GJ. Diagnosis and staging of hepatocellular carcinoma. *Gastroenterology.* 2004;127(suppl 1):S126-S132.
7. Shiina S, Teratani T, Obi S, et al. A randomized controlled trial of radiofrequency ablation with ethanol injection for small hepatocellular carcinoma. *Gastroenterology.* 2005;129:122-130.

I Was Asked to See a Patient With Tense Ascites. How Much Ascites Is Safe to Remove at Any One Time?

Adil Habib, MD
HoChong S. Gilles, MS, FNP
Leslie M. Gallagher, MS, ANP
Douglas M. Heuman, MD

Therapeutic paracentesis plays a crucial role in managing symptoms and preventing complications of tense ascites. We believe strongly that there is no limit to the volume of fluid that can be removed safely during a paracentesis, provided the procedure is performed properly. The small risk of postparacentesis circulatory dysfunction (PPCD) leading to renal failure is largely eliminated by concurrent administration of albumin and meticulous sterile technique. In our view, the more timid approach of limited paracentesis is associated with a greater risk of complications because of the persistent large fluid burden and the need for more frequent abdominal punctures.

The problems associated with tense ascites are not just cosmetic. Pressure on the diaphragm produces restrictive pulmonary physiology and dyspnea and predisposes to atelectasis and pneumonia. Peritoneal tension is associated with anorexia and early satiety, and the resulting malnutrition may lead to a vicious cycle of impaired hepatic synthetic function, declining serum albumin, and prerenal azotemia with aggravation of salt retention and hyponatremia. Malnutrition is also associated with impaired immune function that predisposes to infectious complications. Transient bacteremias may lead to infection of ascites, resulting in spontaneous bacterial peritonitis. Increased abdominal wall tension combined with weakening of muscle and connective tissue from malnutrition leads to painful umbilical and inguinal hernias that may incarcerate or spontaneously rupture. The sheer weight of the ascites may limit the patient's mobility, leading to deconditioning. Tense ascites increases the hepatic venous pressure gradient, intravariceal pressure, and variceal wall tension and may predispose to variceal hemorrhage.

Given the obvious benefits of ascites decompression, it is unfortunate that many physicians are reluctant to perform therapeutic paracentesis. The basis of this reluctance dates to physiological studies carried out in the 1960s indicating that ascites could reform rapidly following therapeutic paracentesis, and this fluid shift could lead to contraction of the circulating volume and occasionally precipitate renal failure. This phenomenon, now termed *postparacentesis circulatory dysfunction syndrome*, is characterized by an increase in sympathetic nervous output accompanied by increased plasma renin activity and aldosterone, peaking after 24 to 48 h. This is often accompanied by increased serum creatinine and hyponatremia. Some degree of PPCD occurs about 15% to 20% of the time following paracentesis in excess of 5 L. Though most cases are mild and asymptomatic and resolve spontaneously, patients who experience PPCD after large volume paracentesis are at increased risk of renal failure and have higher 30-day mortality.

While PPCD is a real phenomenon, it is important to appreciate two facts about this condition. First, it is most likely to occur in patients whose livers have already reached an advanced stage of terminal decompensation, and the poor prognosis may relate more to the underlying disease than to the acute effects of paracentesis. Second, it can largely be prevented even in very sick patients by concurrent administration of human serum albumin. Quintero and colleagues in Barcelona were the first to demonstrate the safety of routine total paracentesis when accompanied by albumin infusion,[1] and this was subsequently confirmed in other large prospective trials. In a study in which cirrhotic patients undergoing therapeutic paracentesis were randomized to receive albumin (10 g/L of ascites removed) or placebo, the incidence of azotemia or hyponatremia following paracentesis was only 3.8% in patients receiving albumin, compared to 20.8% in controls.[2] Albumin was found to be more effective than dextran 70, polygeline, or saline for preventing PPCD.[3]

Although the practice of administering albumin to patients undergoing large volume paracentesis has become almost universal among hepatologists, it does have its critics. They point out correctly that albumin has not been proven to affect survival following large volume paracentesis. Some features of PPCD such as decreased peripheral vascular resistance cannot easily be attributed to a decreased intravascular volume and may not be reversible with albumin. Excessive albumin infusion can cause pulmonary edema. Albumin is expensive and the supply is limited. Finally, there is no solid evidence on which to base a recommendation regarding how much albumin to give. Some algorithms call for administration of 6 to 8 g of albumin per liter of ascites removed; others routinely give a fixed infusion of 50 g of albumin. We prefer the latter approach, which is in line with recent practice guidelines.[4]

On the other side of the equation, some complications actually may be less common with total paracentesis than with limited paracentesis. Each paracentesis is associated with a small but unavoidable risk of intraperitoneal hemorrhage from puncture of an abdominal wall varix; the more ascites is removed at the initial paracentesis, the fewer subsequent paracenteses should be required. Persistent leakage of ascites fluid from the puncture site is less likely following total than partial paracentesis. Because ascites may reaccumulate rapidly, limited paracentesis gives only transitory relief and in our experience is relatively ineffective for managing the nutritional and other complications associated with tense ascites.

The technique employed in performing total paracentesis is important. We choose an optimal site in the lateral right or left lower quadrant using bedside ultrasound to minimize risk of perforating bowel or lacerating liver or spleen. Sterile technique must be maintained, as seeding of ascites with bacteria may lead to peritonitis. Because it is difficult to preserve an aseptic field if the procedure is prolonged, speed is of some importance. We use disposable paracentesis kits with a blunt trochar/stylet and with sterile tubing matched to a peristaltic pump (GI Supply). This system allows continuous withdrawal of fluid into easily disposable 2-L plastic bags at adjustable rates up to 20 L per hour. We routinely administer intravenous albumin while the ascites fluid is being withdrawn.

In our practice almost all large volume paracenteses today are performed on an outpatient basis by a trained and experienced hepatology nurse practitioner, rather than by physicians, whose services are in great demand elsewhere. Since we adopted this policy 6 years ago, admissions for management of ascites have decreased dramatically and complications of paracentesis have become rare. We routinely remove all mobilizable ascites when we perform a therapeutic paracentesis. The largest volume we have removed at one sitting was 29 L, and our average over the last 600 procedures was 11 L per session; the average time required is under 1 hour and no session has lasted longer than 2 h. Treatment is very accessible, usually available on demand within 1 working day, and patient satisfaction is very high.

References

1. Quintero E, Gines P, Arroyo V, et al. Paracentesis versus diuretics in the treatment of cirrhotics with tense ascites. *Lancet.* 1985;1:611-612.
2. Gines P, Tito L, Arroyo V, et al. Randomized comparative study of therapeutic paracentesis with and without intravenous albumin in cirrhosis. *Gastroenterology.* 1988;94:1493-1502.
3. Gines A, Fernandez-Esparrach G, Monescillo A, et al. Randomized trial comparing albumin, Dextran 70, and polygeline in cirrhotic patients with ascites treated by paracentesis. *Gastroenterology.* 1996;111:1002-1010.
4. Runyon BA. Management of adult patients with ascites due to cirrhosis. *Hepatology.* 2004;39:841-856.

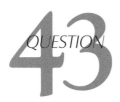
I Have Been Increasing the Dose of Diuretics in My Patient With Ascites Over Several Weeks. He Still Has Ascites but Has Now Developed an Elevation in Serum Creatinine to 2.0 mg/dL. What Should I Do?

Douglas M. Heuman, MD
Adil Habib, MD

Rising creatinine in the cirrhotic patient with ascites is a potentially ominous finding. It requires immediate attention to identify and address the underlying cause. Six possible explanations should be considered in this situation.

First, azotemia may simply reflect overaggressive diuresis of cirrhotic ascites. Studies in the 1960s by Gabuzda and colleagues demonstrated that the maximum rate of absorption of ascites from the peritoneum is on the order of 500 mL per day.[1] While peripheral edema is present, diuresis can proceed rapidly, since tissue fluid can be mobilized quickly. Once edema has cleared, however, continued aggressive diuresis may lead to significant contraction of the circulating volume with reduced renal perfusion and prerenal azotemia. Cessation of diuretics, perhaps with a brief infusion of saline or albumin, usually will reverse the azotemia, after which diuretics can be resumed at a lower dose.

Second, the patient's ascites may not be due to cirrhosis. Not all ascites in the cirrhotic patient is cirrhotic ascites. Patients with cirrhosis may develop ascites for other reasons, including nephrotic syndrome, congestive heart failure, hypothyroidism, chronic pancreatitis, tuberculosis, or malignancy. Current guidelines recommend that a diagnostic paracentesis be performed at the time that ascites first becomes manifest.[2] Cirrhotic ascites is characterized by a low total protein concentration with serum-ascites albumin gradient (SAAG) greater than 1.1 g/dL; if paracentesis confirms this picture, then further diagnostic evaluation usually is unnecessary. Ascites fluids with high protein content and low SAAG reflect exudative processes such as cancer or infection; ascites in these conditions typically does not resolve with diuretic therapy. Treatment should be addressed at the underlying disease, with palliative large volume paracentesis as needed.

Third, a renal insult may have occurred. Cirrhotics are particularly susceptible to nephrotoxicity of nonsteroidal antiinflammatory drugs; these should be sought out and discontinued. Oral neomycin given for suppression of encephalopathy can be absorbed across the cirrhotic gut in sufficient quantities to cause renal failure. Intravenous contrast given for liver imaging studies (computed tomography, angiography) may contribute. Cirrhotics may also have intrinsic renal disease, either related to the cause of their liver disease (immune complex glomerulonephritis in hepatitis B or C, diabetic nephropathy in nonalcoholic steatohepatitis) or due to unrelated conditions such as multiple myeloma. The possibility of obstructive nephropathy from nephrolithiasis, prostatic hypertrophy, or urinary tract cancers also should be considered. Indicators suggestive of intrinsic renal disease include a high fractional excretion of sodium or the finding of leukocytes, blood, or protein on urinalysis. Imaging of the kidneys, ureters, and bladder with ultrasound or computed tomography (CT) and measurement of a postvoid residual may be indicated if obstruction is suspected.

Fourth, the patient's renal perfusion may be compromised by hypotension resulting from infection or hemorrhage. In particular, spontaneous bacterial peritonitis may present insidiously as deterioration of renal function in the cirrhotic patient. Absorption of endotoxin aggravates the generalized vasodilatation of cirrhosis and leads to reduced renal perfusion. Other findings supporting a diagnosis of infection include fever, abdominal pain, deterioration of liver function, and elevation of circulating white blood cells above the patient's baseline. If there is any question of infection, the patient should undergo diagnostic paracentesis, as well as culture of blood and urine, and antibiotic therapy should be initiated. The patient should also be given albumin to expand the circulating volume; this measure is effective in preventing progressive renal failure in patients with spontaneous bacterial peritonitis.[3]

Fifth, the patient's ascites may have become refractory to medical therapy. The term *refractory ascites* is reserved for cases in which either (a) ascites persists despite maximal therapy with diuretics and salt restriction, or (b) ascites persists because patients cannot tolerate maximal diuretic therapy secondary to development of azotemia or hyponatremia.[4] Refractory ascites occurs in 5% to 10% of all patients with cirrhosis and is a poor prognostic sign, indicative of impending terminal decompensation; at least 50% will die within 1 year. If accompanied by hyponatremia or azotemia, the prognosis is even worse. Management options include liver transplantation, serial large volume paracentesis (LVP), transjugular intrahepatic portasystemic shunt (TIPS), or peritoneovenous shunt.[5] Of these, only liver transplantation has been shown to improve survival. TIPS may be useful for mobilizing ascites in patients with well-preserved hepatic function but risks aggravating hepatic encephalopathy.[6] Large volume paracentesis provides palliative benefit and usually will not aggravate azotemia, provided that the patient receives intravenous albumin concurrently (see Question 42).

Sixth and finally, the patient may be developing hepatorenal syndrome. This serious complication of end-stage liver disease occurs almost exclusively in patients with ascites. It is characterized by renal cortical vasospasm and reduced glomerular filtration rate with elevated serum creatinine. Fractional excretion of sodium is low. The condition fails to normalize with volume expansion. The underlying trigger appears to be an extreme renal cortical vasospasm in response to systemic vasodilatation with hypotension, as well as unknown circulating vasoactive toxins. Two general patterns are recognized. Type II hepatorenal syndrome is characterized by persistent stable creatinine elevation that may persist for many months; creatinine clearance may fluctuate with changes in circulating volume but does not normalize. Type I hepatorenal syndrome is characterized by hypotension and rapidly progressive azotemia with oliguria, leading to uremia; unless it can be reversed immediately, patients usually die within weeks. Type II hepatorenal syndrome is managed as refractory ascites. Type I hepatorenal syndrome can sometimes be corrected by aggressive intervention with volume expansion (typically albumin), vasoconstrictors (midodrine plus octreotide, terlipressin, norepinephrine drip), as well as antibiotics. If these measures fail, urgent liver transplantation is required. Hemodialysis may be useful as a bridge to transplantation.

In a case such as the one described, we would discontinue diuretics. We would send urine for sodium, creatinine, and urinalysis and would also send blood for liver tests, electrolytes, complete blood count, and coagulation studies. We might give an intravenous infusion of saline or albumin. If history and physical showed no sign of infection or deteriorating liver function, we would consider outpatient management with frequent follow-up (generally at daily intervals until clear improvement is seen). However, if there is evidence of infection or deteriorating liver function, or if the patient's renal function fails to respond immediately to these conservative measures, we would hospitalize for further diagnostic evaluation and therapy.

Any patient with cirrhotic ascites, particularly one who has experienced azotemia, should be evaluated for liver transplantation.[7] If no contraindication to transplantation is identified, the patient should be referred to a transplant center for listing. Creatinine is one of the components of the model for end-stage liver disease (MELD), the prognostic model used to allocate organs for liver transplantation in the United States.[8] Cirrhotic patients with significant azotemia usually have high MELD scores and receive high priority for transplantation.

References

1. Shear L, Ching S, Gabuzda GJ. Compartmentalization of ascites and edema in patients with hepatic cirrhosis. *N Engl J Med.* 1970;282:1391-1396.
2. Runyon BA. Management of adult patients with ascites due to cirrhosis. *Hepatology.* 2004;39:841-856.
3. Bass NM. Intravenous albumin for spontaneous bacterial peritonitis in patients with cirrhosis. *N Engl J Med.* 1999;341:443-444.
4. Arroyo V, Gines P, Gerbes AL, et al. Definition and diagnostic criteria of refractory ascites and hepatorenal syndrome in cirrhosis. International Ascites Club. *Hepatology.* 1996;23:164-176.
5. Moore KP, Wong F, Gines P, et al. The management of ascites in cirrhosis: report on the consensus conference of the International Ascites Club. *Hepatology.* 2003;38:258-266.
6. Sanyal AJ, Genning C, Reddy KR, et al. The North American Study for the Treatment of Refractory Ascites. *Gastroenterology.* 2003;124:634-641.

7. Murray KF, Carithers RL Jr. AASLD practice guidelines: Evaluation of the patient for liver transplantation. *Hepatology.* 2005;41:1407-1432.
8. Kamath PS, Kim WR. The model for end-stage liver disease (MELD). *Hepatology.* 2007;45:797-805.

44

MY PATIENT WITH CRYPTOGENIC CIRRHOSIS WAS RECENTLY HOSPITALIZED WITH SPONTANEOUS BACTERIAL PERITONITIS. HOW LONG SHOULD SHE BE TREATED WITH ANTIBIOTICS?

Paul Arnold, MD
Adil Habib, MD
Douglas M. Heuman, MD

Spontaneous bacterial peritonitis (SBP) is a potentially lethal infection in the cirrhotic patient. It should be sought aggressively and treated early with effective antibiotics. The duration of treatment is dictated by the results of cultures, severity of illness, and clinical response to therapy. Any patient who has experienced SBP is at high risk to recur and should receive long-term prophylactic antibiotic therapy for as long as ascites persists.

SBP occurs commonly in the setting of cirrhotic ascites. Two pathophysiological factors are at work.[1] First, cirrhotic ascites fluid is a good culture medium because it is transudative in nature, with a very low protein concentration. Thus, concentrations of antibacterial proteins such as immunoglobulins and complement are low. When bacteria gain access to the ascites, they are able to proliferate rapidly. Second, cirrhotic patients frequently experience transient bacteremias, because portal hypertension predisposes to translocation of enteric bacteria across the enteric mucosa, and because portosystemic shunts allow these bacteria to escape phagocytosis by the hepatic Kupffer cells. Other sources of bacteremia such as pneumonia, urinary tract infection, or indwelling cannulas also can lead to SBP, and direct seeding of the peritoneum can occur during paracentesis if sterile technique is not strictly observed. Patients with ascites who experience variceal hemorrhage are at particularly high risk to develop SBP.

The classical presentation of SBP is a patient with cirrhotic ascites who develops abdominal pain over hours to days, usually of moderate severity, accompanied by fever and peripheral blood leukocytosis. However, atypical presentations lacking these features are very common. SBP may present as exacerbation of hepatic encephalopathy, deterioration of liver function, or worsening azotemia and hyponatremia. Many cases of SBP are detected at a completely asymptomatic stage by analysis of ascites fluid removed during therapeutic paracentesis.

When SBP is suspected, a diagnostic paracentesis usually should be performed urgently and sent for cell count and differential as well as for aerobic and anaerobic culture. An ascites fluid neutrophil count greater than 250 is suspicious for SBP, and a neutrophil count exceeding 500 is considered diagnostic.[2] Cultures may be negative in nearly half of SBP cases. Yield may improve if ascites fluid is inoculated directly into a blood culture bottle at the bedside at the time of paracentesis. Urine culture and paired blood cultures should be obtained as well; these have lower yield but will sometimes provide an etiological diagnosis when ascites cultures are negative. Urinalysis and chest X-ray are useful for excluding other common infections.

SBP must be distinguished from secondary bacterial peritonitis caused by intra-abdominal surgical emergencies such as appendicitis. Patients with secondary peritonitis usually are quite sick, with severe abdominal pain and guarding, very high levels of leukocytes in ascites fluid, and polymicrobial infection including anaerobic bacteria.[3] If secondary peritonitis is suspected, emergent abdominal imaging and surgical consultation should be obtained.

Early antimicrobial therapy is critical in the management of patients with SBP. The initial choice of antibitotics is directed toward the most likely pathogens. Enteric gram-negative rods such as *Escherichia coli* and *Klebsiella pneumoniae* are responsible for about three fourths of cases of SBP. Less common causes include pneumococcus, enterococcus, other streptococcal species, staphylococcus, anaerobes, and fungi. Choice of antibiotics must take into account the evolving spectrum of microbial resistance in the community as well as patient-specific factors such as prior antibiotic treatment or likely source of infection (for example, staphylococcal coverage in patients who develop SBP within 1 week following a therapeutic paracentesis). Currently we prefer to initiate treatment with a third-generation cephalosporin such as ceftriaxone while awaiting culture data. If the patient is critically ill, we also add vancomycin and metronidazole. Other reasonable choices of antimicrobial agents include imipenem, aztreonam, ampicillin-sulbactam, ticarcillin-clavulanate, amoxicillin-clavulanic acid, and the fluoroquinolones.[4]

Patients with suspected SBP should be given intravenous albumin to expand plasma volume. Absorption of bacterial endotoxins into the circulation of the cirrhotic patient causes vasodilatation, hypotension, and reduced renal perfusion and can precipitate hepatorenal syndrome. Intravenous albumin, initiated at the same time antibiotic therapy is started, helps to maintain renal perfusion and has been shown to reduce risk of renal failure and death.[5]

If cultures of blood or ascites fluid demonstrate the causative organism, antimicrobial therapy should be adjusted to optimize coverage. For milder infections, including those caused by common gram negatives and those that are culture negative, we often switch to oral antibiotics and complete an outpatient course of treatment.[6] In more severe cases, especially those with positive blood cultures, or cases caused by hard-to-treat organisms such as staphylococcus or enterococcus, we continue intravenous antibiotics and observe in hospital until the infection has come under control, as documented by clearing of pain and fever, stabilization of liver function, and normalization of ascites fluid leukocyte counts on follow-up paracentesis. In routine cases, if a follow-up paracentesis after 5 days of treatment shows normalization of the leukocyte count, treatment can be discontinued safely.[7] Longer courses may be required for hard-to-treat organisms, especially if bacteremia is documented. Current literature does not permit firm recommendations with regard to duration of therapy,[4] so we tend to err on the side of conservatism.

As many as 90% of patients who have experienced an episode of SBP will experience another episode within 1 year, unless prophylactic measures are taken. Antimicrobial prophylaxis has been shown to reduce the annual risk of SBP recurrence to less than 20%.[8,9] Daily administration of norfloxacin or other quinolones appears to be the most effective prophylactic regimen. Sulfamethoxazole-trimethoprim given 5 times weekly was also effective in early studies but appears to be losing efficacy as bacterial resistance evolves. Once-weekly ciprofloxacin also reduces SBP recurrence, but this regimen is probably less effective than daily ciprofloxacin and may be associated with a higher risk of resistance. When a patient on prophylaxis does develop SBP, the responsible organism is usually resistant to the antibiotic that had been given for prophylaxis, and this must be taken into account in choosing empirical coverage.

Since the risk of SBP is eliminated by controlling ascites, patients with SBP tend to be individuals whose ascites is refractory to medical therapy. Such patients have advanced cirrhosis and a poor long-term prognosis. This is why 1-year mortality following an episode of SBP exceeds 50%. Transjugular intrahepatic portosystemic shunting in selected patients with well-preserved liver function may improve diuretic response and allow ascites to resolve, but it does not appear to alter survival. We recommend continuing prophylaxis until and unless ascites resolves completely. Liver transplantation should be considered in all cirrhotic patients who have experienced an episode of SBP.

References

1. Wong F, Bernardi M, Balk R, et al. Sepsis in cirrhosis: report on the 7th meeting of the International Ascites Club. *Gut*. 2005;54:718-725.
2. Runyon BA. The evolution of ascitic fluid analysis in the diagnosis of spontaneous bacterial peritonitis. *Am J Gastroenterol*. 2003;98:1675-1677.
3. Gomez-Jimenez J, Ribera E, Gasser I, Pahissa A, Martinez-Vazquez JM. Differentiation of spontaneous from secondary bacterial peritonitis in cirrhotics. *Gastroenterology*. 1990;99:1538-1540.
4. Soares-Weiser K, Brezis M, Leibovici L. Antibiotics for spontaneous bacterial peritonitis in cirrhotics. *Cochrane Database Syst Rev*. 2001;No. 3:CD002232.
5. Bass NM. Intravenous albumin for spontaneous bacterial peritonitis in patients with cirrhosis. *N Engl J Med*. 1999;341:443-444.
6. Ricart E, Soriano G, Novella MT, et al. Amoxicillin-clavulanic acid versus cefotaxime in the therapy of bacterial infections in cirrhotic patients. *J Hepatol*. 2000;32:596-602.
7. Franca A, Giordano HM, Seva-Pereira T, Soares EC. Five days of ceftriaxone to treat spontaneous bacterial peritonitis in cirrhotic patients. *J Gastroenterol*. 2002;37:119-122.
8. Gines P, Navasa M. Antibiotic prophylaxis for spontaneous bacterial peritonitis: how and whom? *J Hepatol*. 1998;29:490-494.
9. Mowat C, Stanley AJ. Review article: spontaneous bacterial peritonitis—diagnosis, treatment and prevention. *Aliment Pharmacol Ther*. 2001;15:1851-1859.

45

MY PATIENT WITH CIRRHOSIS HAS AN ELEVATED SERUM AMMONIA BUT NO SYMPTOMS OF HEPATIC ENCEPHALOPATHY. HOW MUCH LACTULOSE SHOULD I RECOMMEND?

Paul Arnold, MD
Adil Habib, MD
Douglas M. Heuman, MD

We do not place much reliance on blood ammonia measurements in the clinical setting. Hepatic encephalopathy is not a biochemical diagnosis but a clinical diagnosis based on history and neuropsychological findings. Ammonia is not the only toxin contributing to encephalopathy; ambient levels of blood ammonia correlate poorly with severity of encephalopathy, and artefactual elevations of ammonia due to improper sample handling are very common. That having been said, cirrhotic patients may have subtle cognitive defects that can escape detection with routine clinical evaluation, and treatment of minimal hepatic encephalopathy seems to improve cognitive function and quality of life in a number of ways.[1] So in the patient described here, further clinical evaluation may be warranted in an effort to identify subtle features of minimal hepatic encephalopathy. If minimal encephalopathy is suspected, then a trial of lactulose is warranted. The dosage of lactulose usually starts at 15 to 30 mL once or twice daily, titrating upwards to achieve between 2 to 4 bowel movements per day.

Hepatic encephalopathy is a condition in which circulating neurotoxins alter brain function, leading to impaired concentration, somnolence, stupor, and coma.[2] The toxins originate mainly in the colon, via action of intestinal bacteria on protein and other dietary components. These toxins normally would be delivered to the liver in the portal blood and cleared before reaching the systemic circulation, but in cirrhosis this clearance fails because of portosystemic shunting. Ammonia has long been considered a key player in hepatic encephalopathy, but the evidence for this is inconclusive. Ammonia is in many respects a likely candidate. It is generated in the colon through bacterial action. Ammonia is neurotoxic, producing astrocytic changes in vitro that resemble the changes seen in the brains of patients with hepatic encephalopathy. Many conditions that increase colonic ammonia generation in cirrhotic patients, such as dietary protein load or constipation, tend to aggravate encephalopathy. Circulating ammonia levels tend to be increased in patients with cirrhosis and encephalopathy, and mean ammonia levels tend to be higher in patients with more severe encephalopathy. Finally, treatments such as lactulose or antibiotics that reduce circulating ammonia appear to be effective in controlling symptoms of encephalopathy.

However, ammonia is not the whole story. Conditions that are associated with pure elevation of blood ammonia, such as hereditary urea cycle defects, produce excitatory changes on electroencephelogram (EEG), seizures, and other findings that are very different from the manifestations of hepatic encephalopathy. Levels of ammonia in the circulation of individual patients with hepatic encephalopathy correlate poorly with mental status. Numerous studies in cirrhotic patients have found that dietary amino acid challenges may cause striking postprandial increases in ammonia without any detectable change in cognitive function. Conversely, acute reduction in ammonia to normal levels does not necessarily lead to immediate clearing of encephalopathy. Finally, a variety of other neurotoxins have been shown to accumulate in cirrhosis and may contribute to the pathogenesis of encephalopathy.[3]

This is not to say that ammonia is unimportant in pathogenesis of encephalopathy, but rather that circulating levels of ammonia at any given moment are a poor indicator of the extent to which cognitive function is impaired. This is unfortunate because it is not easy to detect and quantify the early stages of hepatic encephalopathy in the clinical setting. Mild encephalopathy is subtle, characterized by such nonspecific symptoms as nighttime insomnia with daytime somnolence, difficulty concentrating, and memory lapses. Neuropsychiatric testing often identifies impairment in motor speed and accuracy, visual perception, visuospatial orientation, visual construction, concentration, attention, and sometimes memory.[4,5] Impairment may be most apparent when patients are faced with complex tasks such as driving. Indeed, recent studies suggest that impaired driving performance on road test simulators is an excellent indicator of minimal hepatic encephalopathy.[6] But neuropsychiatric testing is difficult to apply accurately in day-to-day clinical practice. Newer automated computer-based tests that measure cognitive performance in a variety of domains show promise but are not yet standardized for use in cirrhosis. Functional brain imaging using techniques such as magnetic resonance spectroscopy and positron emission tomography can identify a number of metabolic abnormalities in brains of patients with hepatic encephalopathy, but the sensitivity and specificity of these findings has not been established.[7]

In the meantime, when faced with a cirrhotic patient who may be encephalopathic, we resort to history. We interview the patient, ideally in the company of a spouse or other close contact. We ask about changes in his ability to function at work and home. Has he been having difficulty reading? Is he having trouble with calculations and other abstract skills? Is job performance slipping? Has he had trouble driving—in particular, has he been involved in an accident or gotten lost? We also ask about erratic actions such as irrational extravagant purchases that may represent a change from their usual behavior. During the interview we look for evidence of lethargy, loss of train of thought, and inability to complete sentences. We may request formal neuropsychiatric testing.[5]

In the absence of clinical signs or symptoms of encephalopathy, we would not routinely start patients on treatment, even if ammonia is elevated. At present there is no evidence that prophylactic therapy can alter the natural history of encephalopathy. If there is clinical suspicion of encephalopathy, we will first look for confounding factors that may be contributing, such as sedative drugs. Once these are eliminated, if symptoms persist we usually attempt a therapeutic trial of lactulose, beginning with 15 to 30 mL twice daily. We advise the patient to increase dosage as required until he notes a change in bowel habits with 2 to 3 loose stools daily. Improvement of symptoms on this regimen is presumptive evidence of encephalopathy. Conversely, failure to improve should raise concern for other neurological processes and trigger further evaluation (see Question 46). We advise patients to avoid high-protein binges, but we do not routinely recommend protein restriction below 100 g daily, which can lead to severe malnutrition when used injudiciously.

References

1. Prasad S, Dhiman RK, Duseja A, Chawla YK, Sharma A, Agarwal R. Lactulose improves cognitive functions and health-related quality of life in patients with cirrhosis who have minimal hepatic encephalopathy. *Hepatology.* 2007;45:549-559.
2. Ferenci P, Lockwood A, Mullen K, Tarter R, Weissenborn K, Blei AT. Hepatic encephalopathy—definition, nomenclature, diagnosis, and quantification: final report of the working party at the 11th World Congresses of Gastroenterology, Vienna, 1998. *Hepatology.* 2002;35:716-721.
3. Jones EA. Ammonia, the GABA neurotransmitter system, and hepatic encephalopathy. *Metab Brain Dis.* 2002;17:275-281.
4. Weissenborn K, Giewekemeyer K, Heidenreich S, Bokemeyer M, Berding G, Ahl B. Attention, memory, and cognitive function in hepatic encephalopathy. *Metab Brain Dis.* 2005;20:359-367.
5. Weissenborn K, Ennen JC, Schomerus H, Ruckert N, Hecker H. Neuropsychological characterization of hepatic encephalopathy. *J Hepatol.* 2001;34:768-773.
6. Wein C, Koch H, Popp B, Oehler G, Schauder P. Minimal hepatic encephalopathy impairs fitness to drive. *Hepatology.* 2004;39:739-745.
7. Weissenborn K, Bokemeyer M, Ahl B, et al. Functional imaging of the brain in patients with liver cirrhosis. *Metab Brain Dis.* 2004;19:269-280.

MY PATIENT WITH HEPATIC ENCEPHALOPATHY CONTINUES TO BE MILDLY CONFUSED DESPITE TAKING LACTULOSE TWICE DAILY AND HAVING MULTIPLE EPISODES OF DIARRHEA DAILY. SHOULD I INCREASE THE DOSE FURTHER?

Douglas M Heuman, MD
Adil Habib, MD

Generally, the answer to this question is "No." Lactulose is an effective treatment for hepatic encephalopathy, but it is not innocuous and should not be used promiscuously. Lactulose dosage should be titrated to produce 2 to 4 loose stools per day. Increasing lactulose beyond this point does little to improve encephalopathy while greatly increasing adverse effects such as dehydration, electrolyte derangements, incontinence, perianal irritation, and skin breakdown. Indeed, the metabolic derangements caused by excessive diarrhea (hypernatremia or hyponatremia, hypokalemia, metabolic acidosis) may worsen symptoms of encephalopathy.

When hepatic encephalopathy is refractory to lactulose, one should consider the possibility that the symptoms may have an alternate cause. The differential diagnosis of persistent cognitive impairment in the patient with liver disease is extensive (Table 46-1). Minimal evaluation of the patient with refractory encephalopathy should include magnetic resonance imaging (MRI) of the brain, as well as blood tests for hypothyroidism, syphilis, vitamin B_{12} deficiency, and other correctable causes of dementia. Neurology consultation for more detailed evaluation may be appropriate. Electroencephalography in hepatic encephalopathy typically shows diffuse slowing; unexpected electroencephelo-

---

Table 46-1

Some Examples of Neurological Causes of Cognitive Impairment That Can Be Mistaken for Hepatic Encephalopathy in Patients With Cirrhosis

- Chronic dementias: Alzheimer's, Lewy body, alcoholic
- Vascular disease with multi-infarct dementia
- Chronic subdural hematoma
- CNS infections: crytococcal meningitis, neurosyphilis
- Epilepsy, especially focal or temporal lobe
- Metabolic disorders: hypoglycemia, hypothyroidism
- Nutritional deficiencies: Wernicke-Korsakoff syndrome due to thiamine deficiency, combined systems disease due to vitamin B12 deficiency
- Osmotic demyelination resulting from rapid correction of hyponatremia
- Substance abuse: cannabis, narcotics, hallucinogens, sedatives
- Psychosis: schizophrenia, bipolar disease, depression

---

gram (EEG) findings such as focal seizure activity may point to an alternative cause of the patient's impairment. Lumbar puncture may be useful to exclude a variety of degenerative and chronic infectious processes.

If conditions other than hepatic encephalopathy have been excluded, one should look for exacerbating factors that can be corrected.[1] Patients frequently are noncompliant with lactulose therapy and this can be addressed through counseling. If patients find the taste of liquid lactulose offensive, use of powdered lactulose may be preferred. Concurrent medications may contribute to encephalopathy in a variety of ways, for example, by direct sedative effects (benzodiazepines), by slowing colonic motility (narcotics), or by inducing dehydration or other metabolic derangements (diuretics); changing these may bring the problem under control. Acute deterioration of encephalopathy often is precipitated by gastrointestinal bleeding or acute infections such as spontaneous bacterial peritonitis.

Finally, if encephalopathy persists, one should consider alternative therapeutic interventions. The nonabsorbable antibiotic rifaximin administered orally appears to be as effective as lactulose for control of encephalopathy and has few side effects.[2] Its principal drawback is its cost. Oral neomycin is less expensive and also effective but can occasionally cause acute renal failure in the cirrhotic patient. Severe restriction of dietary protein should be avoided because it leads to protein calorie malnutrition that increases the risk of infection and other complications. Indeed, malnutrition caused by inappropriate protein starvation may produce symptoms of lethargy and listlessness that can be mistaken for encephalopathy. Proteins of vegetable origin may be better tolerated than animal proteins. In the rare patient who cannot ingest 60 to 100 g of protein per day without becoming encephalopathic, one may consider providing specialized nutritional supplements such as Hepaticaid, which are enriched with branched chain amino acids, though these are expensive and of dubious efficacy.[3] Occasionally a patient's symptoms of encephalopathy may be attributable to a large portosystemic shunt, either spontaneous or therapeutic; closure of the shunt by surgical or radiological intervention may ameliorate the encephalopathy.

The definitive treatment of hepatic encephalopathy is liver transplantation. Early referral to a transplant center is encouraged. Unfortunately, hepatic encephalopathy, despite its profound effects on quality of life,[4] does not currently constitute an indication for expedited transplantation,[5] and encephalopathic patients whose liver function is otherwise well compensated may wait years for transplantation under the current system of deceased donor organ allocation. Living donor liver transplantation, which offers a means of circumventing the waiting list, may be an attractive alternative for such patients.

References

1. Ferenci P, Lockwood A, Mullen K, Tarter R, Weissenborn K, Blei AT. Hepatic encephalopathy—definition, nomenclature, diagnosis, and quantification: final report of the working party at the 11th World Congresses of Gastroenterology, Vienna, 1998. *Hepatology.* 2002;35:716-721.
2. Mas A, Rodes J, Sunyer L, et al. Comparison of rifaximin and lactitol in the treatment of acute hepatic encephalopathy: results of a randomized, double-blind, double-dummy, controlled clinical trial. *J Hepatol.* 2003;38:51-58.
3. Is-Nielsen B, Koretz RL, Kjaergard LL, Gluud C. Branched-chain amino acids for hepatic encephalopathy. *Cochrane Database Syst Rev.* 2003;No. 2:CD001939.
4. Prasad S, Dhiman RK, Duseja A, Chawla YK, Sharma A, Agarwal R. Lactulose improves cognitive functions and health-related quality of life in patients with cirrhosis who have minimal hepatic encephalopathy. *Hepatology.* 2007;45:549-559.
5. Ham J, Gish RG, Mullen K. Model for end-stage liver disease (MELD) exception for hepatic encephalopathy. *Liver Transpl.* 2006;12(suppl 3):S102-S104.

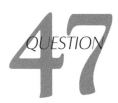

MY PATIENT WITH CIRRHOSIS SUFFERS FROM SEVERE FATIGUE BUT HAS NORMAL LIVER FUNCTION AND HAS NEVER HAD A MAJOR COMPLICATION OF CIRRHOSIS. SHOULD I REFER THIS PATIENT FOR A LIVER TRANSPLANT?

Amrita Sethi, MD
R. Todd Stravitz, MD

No. In the absence of complications of cirrhosis, fatigue in a cirrhotic patient is not an indication for referral for liver transplant evaluation.

One of the most important decisions facing a physician caring for a patient with cirrhosis is when to refer for consideration of liver transplantation. In general, patients with normal liver chemistries and without major complications of cirrhosis do not require referral because they have an excellent short-term prognosis. However, they should be under the care of a physician with training in liver disease, for inexperience may lead to a late referral for consideration of liver transplantation, jeopardizing a patient's ability to undergo a successful transplant.

Based upon extensive data on the natural history of cirrhosis, the patient presenting with compensated, uncomplicated cirrhosis has a nearly 100% 3-month survival. Therefore, liver transplant evaluation would clearly be inappropriate, considering that the liver transplant procedure itself carries about a 10% 3-month mortality. However, the appearance of complications of cirrhosis, such as recurrent variceal bleeding, ascites, hepatic hydrothorax, azotemia, and hepatic encephalopathy, should trigger referral to a transplant center because they are associated with increased short-term mortality (Table 47-1).

Prior to 2002, the Child-Turcotte-Pugh (CTP) score was widely used for estimating short-term mortality in patents with cirrhosis and formed the basis for assigning priority

Table 47-1

Indications for Referral of a Patient With Cirrhosis to a Liver Transplant Center for Evaluation

1. First complication of cirrhosis
- Ascites/hydrothorax
- Hepatic encephalopathy
- Azotemia
- Variceal bleed
2. Child-Turcotte-Pugh (CTP) score ≥7[†]
3. Model for end-stage liver disease (MELD) score ≥10
4. Suspicion of hepatocellular carcinoma
   - Mass on abdominal imaging
   - Rising alpha-fetoprotein
5. Consideration of alternative therapies

*Adapted from Stravitz.[1]
[†]The CTP score is calculated as described in Table 47-2. The MELD score is calculated as $3.8 \cdot \log_e$ (bilirubin [mg/dL] + $11.2 \cdot \log_e$ (INR) + $9.6 \cdot \log_e$ (creatinine [mg/dL]), or online at: www.mayo.edu/int-med/gi/model/mayomodl.htm

to receive a liver transplant in patients on the transplant waiting list (Table 47-2). The CTP score is calculated by assigning 1 to 3 points for the severity of hepatic encephalopathy and ascites, as well as deviation from the normal range of albumin, prothrombin time, and bilirubin. Liver transplant evaluation was often undertaken in patients with cirrhosis and CTP scores of 7 or higher. Several features of the CTP score, however, made the system unfair and insufficiently accurate in predicting short-term mortality, including the subjectivity of assessing the severity of ascites and encephalopathy.

Consequently, the CTP scheme for prioritizing patients awaiting liver transplantation was replaced in 2002 by the model for end-stage liver disease (MELD) score, an empirically derived calculation originally used to estimate 3-month mortality of patients undergoing transjugular intrahepatic shunt (TIPS) placement. MELD did away with subjective parameters of ascites and encephalopathy and considers only objective laboratory parameters: total bilirubin, creatinine, and INR. Subsequent studies have demonstrated the superiority of MELD over CTP in predicting 3-month mortality. MELD scores range from 6 to 40 points, with 3-month mortalities of about 2% for a score less than 9 to 70% for a score greater than 40, but occasionally can go higher (Figure 47-1). A MELD of 10 has been advocated by some authorities as an indication for liver transplant evaluation. However, patients are not activated on the liver transplant waiting list until their MELD scores approach 15, the point at which 3-month mortality without transplant equals the 3-month mortality of the transplant (ie, 10%).

Referral for liver transplant evaluation should also seriously be considered in any patient with cirrhosis who develops a mass on abdominal imaging suggestive of hepatocellular carcinoma (HCC). Liver transplantation has become the most effective therapy for HCC in patients with cirrhosis, and long-term, tumor-free survival approaches that of

Table 47-2

Modified Child-Turcotte-Pugh (CTP) Score for Assessing Severity of Liver Failure

Feature	1 Point	2 Points	3 Points
Encephalopathy	0	+	++
Ascites	0	+	++
Bilirubin (mg/dL)	<2.0	2 to 3	>3.0
Albumin (g/dL)	>3.5	2.8 to 3.5	<2.8
Prothrombin time (seconds prolonged)	1 to 4	4 to 6	>6

CTP Score*	3-Month Mortality, %[†]
<7-9	4.3
10-12	11.2
13-15	40.1

*A total score of 5 to 6 points correlates to CTP class A, 7 to 9 points to class B, and 10 to 15 points to class C.
[†]Data from Wiesner et al.[4]

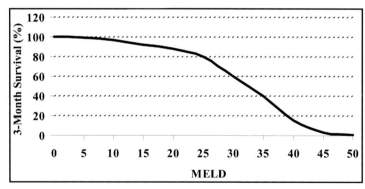

Figure 47-1. Estimated 3-month survival in patients with cirrhosis according to MELD score. Adapted from Wiesner R, Edwards E, Freeman R, et al. Model for end-stage liver disease (MELD) and allocation of donor livers. *Gastroenterology.* 2003; 124:91-96.

transplant recipients without malignancy provided that tumor stage is limited. In community hospitals, the diagnosis of HCC in a patient with cirrhosis is hampered by a lack of mutlidisciplinary expertise. Therefore, most patients without extensive disease should be considered for referral to a liver transplant center.

A final indication for referral to a liver transplant center in patients with compensated cirrhosis is to consider alternative therapies for the underlying liver disease that carry risk of hepatic decompensation. The most common clinical situation is to consider antiviral therapy in a patient with cirrhosis due to hepatitis C, which carries a small but not insignificant risk of severe complications. Such patients with marginal liver reserve may be best served by early liver transplant evaluation in anticipation of the need for urgent transplantation during antiviral therapy.

In summary, the patient presented does not meet any of the criteria for referral for transplant evaluation discussed above. While many patients with cirrhosis complain of incapacitating fatigue, the symptom is nonspecific and does not predict short-term mortality, which remains the litmus test by which patients receive priority for liver transplantation.

References

1. Stravitz, RT. Management of the cirrhotic patient before liver transplantation: the role of the referring gastro-enterologist. *Gastroenterol Hepatol.* 2006;2:346-354.
2. Murray KF, Carithers RL Jr. AASLD practice guidelines: evaluation of the patient for liver transplantation. *Hepatology.* 2005;41:1407-1432.
3. Kamath PS, Wiesner RH, Malinchoc M, et al. A model to predict survival in patients with end-stage liver disease. *Hepatology.* 2001;33:464-470.
4. Wiesner R, Edwards E, Freeman R, et al. Model for end-stage liver disease (MELD) and allocation of donor livers. *Gastroenterology.* 2003;124:91-96.

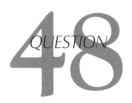

48

WHAT SHOULD I RECOMMEND FOR MY PATIENT WITH CIRRHOSIS WHO WAS RECENTLY FOUND TO HAVE A NEW 2-CENTIMETER LIVER MASS BY ULTRASOUND SCREENING?

Lawrence Chang, MD
R. Todd Stravitz, MD

In a patient with cirrhosis, the differential diagnosis of a new liver mass found on ultrasound (US) surveillance includes malignant and nonmalignant macronodules. Hepatocellular carcinoma (HCC) is obviously the primary concern. Major risk factors for developing HCC in patients with cirrhosis include older age, male sex, a family history of HCC, coinfection with more than one hepatotropic virus (hepatitis B and C), and coinfection with human immunodeficiency virus (HIV). The risk of developing HCC in a patient with cirrhosis varies with the etiology of underlying liver disease, with highest risk in patients with active hepatitis B and C viral replication (3% to 5%/year). However, the risk of HCC is probably increased in any patient with cirrhosis regardless of underlying liver disease. Nonmalignant macronodules in patients with cirrhosis include large regenerative, and low-grade and high-grade dysplastic nodules. Although the malignant potential of nonmalignant macronodules including regenerative nodules is debated, prospective studies suggest that high-grade dysplastic nodules may increase the risk of developing HCC at least 4.5-fold in patients with cirrhosis. Therefore, the appearance of any new solid lesion on surveillance US in a patient with cirrhosis is concerning.

Surveillance for HCC in patients with cirrhosis has been widely advocated with the preheld conviction that earlier diagnosis would lead to better survival. However, the wide adoption of surveillance programs has precluded randomized, prospective studies to demonstrate proof of this concept. In the era of liver transplantation, however, several

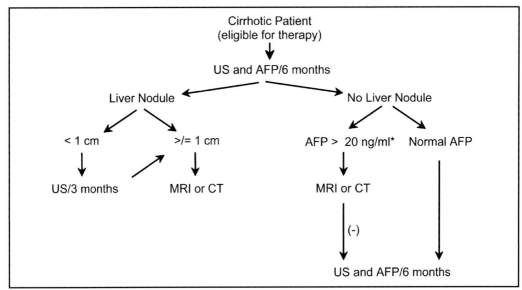

Figure 48-1. Surveillance algorithm for HCC in patients with cirrhosis. The cut-off for AFP in patients without nodules on US where further abdominal imaging should be considered has not been defined. The suggestion of 20 ng/ml may be appropriate for patients with non-viral chronic liver disease, and higher for patients with chronic active hepatitis B or C (Adapted from Bruix J, Sherman M, Llovet JM, et al. Clinical management of hepatocellular carcinoma. Conclusions of the Barcelona-2000 EASL conference. European Association for the Study of the Liver. *J Hepatol.* 2001;35:421-430).

studies have suggested that surveillance increases the opportunity to diagnose HCC earlier so that transplant may be safely performed with minimal risk of recurrence. The mode of surveillance in a known cirrhotic should be by US performed by an experienced radiologist, and the interval of surveillance should be every 6 months, although one large study suggested that surveillance every 12 months was as effective as every 6 months in detecting early stage tumors. Surveillance should be limited to patients who are eligible for therapy of HCC (Figure 48-1).

The use of alpha-fetoprotein (AFP) in surveillance for HCC in patients with cirrhosis is controversial. Unquestionably, the test lacks sensitivity and specificity; at a cut-off of 20 ng/mL, the sensitivity of AFP is only 60%, and positive predictive value assuming a 5% prevalence of HCC is only around 40%. The specificity of elevated AFP varies with the etiology of underlying liver disease and is especially low in patients with active hepatitis B or hepatitis C replication. However, the test is useful in confirming a diagnosis of HCC in a patient with a liver mass if markedly elevated (>200 ng/mL) or increasing on serial determinations. In a patient with a negative US but AFP > 20 ng/mL, further abdominal imaging may be therefore be considered, especially in patients with cirrhosis from a non-viral etiology (Figure 48-1).

The appearance of any new solid lesion >1 cm on US surveillance mandates the performance of more sensitive and specific imaging studies (Figure 48-1). Gadolinium-enhanced magnetic resonance imaging (MRI) or triple-phase contrast-enhanced computed tomography (CT) serve this purpose equally well and should be the next test for the patient presented, depending upon the expertise of the local radiologist. The importance of radi-

---

Table 48-1

Diagnostic Criteria for HCC in Patients With Cirrhosis According to the European Association for the Study of Liver Disease*

Diagnostic Criteria for HCC

Compatible histology, **OR**

Radiologic criteria: Serologic criteria:

Lesion >2 cm with arterial enhancement Two coincident
imaging techniques, OR[†]

Lesion >2 cm with arterial enhancement One imaging   AFP >400 ng/mL[‡]
technique

*Adapted from Bruix J, Sherman M, Llovet JM, et al. Clinical management of hepatocellular carcinoma. Conclusions of the Barcelona-2000 EASL conference. European Association for the Study of the Liver. *J Hepatol.* 2001;35:421-430
[†]Abdominal imaging techniques include US, CT, MRI, and angiography.
[‡]Subsequent studies have suggested an AFP of 200 ng/mL.

---

ologist and technician experience with these imaging modalities cannot be overstated, because the proper timing of intravenous contrast and image acquisition is crucial for the detection and characterization of mass lesions in a cirrhotic liver. A peculiarity of HCC is its development of a blood supply from the hepatic artery, in contrast to the nonmalignant surrounding liver, which derives most of its blood supply from the portal vein. Therefore, HCC classically enhances in the hepatic arterial phase but becomes relatively hypointense in the portal venous phase of contrast administration (so-called "early washout"). Indeed, cirrhotic patients with lesions of >2 cm and these enhancement characteristics on two imaging modalities can be reliably diagnosed with HCC without the need for biopsy (Table 48-1). The presence of an AFP of >200 ng/mL and arterial enhancement on one imaging study is also diagnostic for HCC without the need for biopsy.

Accordingly, the role of biopsy in diagnosing HCC in patients with cirrhosis has diminished with improvements in abdominal imaging techniques. Biopsy should be reserved for liver masses in non-cirrhotic livers, in whom the probability of HCC is lower, and should be considered in cirrhotic patients with lesions of 1 to 2 cm or where enhancement characteristics are nondiagnostic on imaging. In practice, however, since HCC of 1 to 2 cm rarely metastasize and biopsy carries risk of bleeding and seeding of malignant cells, many experts would repeat the advanced imaging study in 3 months to look for enlargement of the lesion.

After confirming a diagnosis of HCC, assessment of disease extension should be considered. The contrast-enhanced abdominal CT or MRI should provide adequate hepatic tumor staging, specifically, the number, size, and location of lesions, as well as the patency of the portal vein. Portal vein thrombosis is an ominous sign of advanced tumor stage since HCC has a predilection to invade portal branches. Duplex ultrasound or MR angiography may be useful adjuncts, but visceral angiography may occasionally be necessary. Extrahepatic spread of HCC usually occurs to the lungs or to bone, and contrast-enhanced chest CT and bone scintigraphy should therefore be performed. In general, patients with metastatic HCC or HCC with portal venous invasion are not candidates for therapy outside of experimental chemotherapeutic trials.

In the absence of extrahepatic disease, the treatment of HCC must be individualized based upon the extent of intrahepatic disease, the severity of liver failure from cirrhosis, the presence of portal hypertension, and consideration of comorbid medical problems. Well-compensated cirrhotic patients with local disease and no evidence of portal hypertension (no esophageal varices, normal platelet counts) may be candidates for surgical resection; however, this clinical scenario is rare in the United States. Much more frequently, the risk of severe decompensation outweighs the possible benefit of resection, and other therapy must be considered. In addition, resection does not cure the premalignant environment of the cirrhotic liver, and 5-year recurrence rates after resection approach 70%.

Since the mid-1990s, the treatment of choice for HCC of limited tumor stage has become liver transplantation (LT), which removes tumor and the premalignant environment and cures the portal hypertension. A seminal study from Milan in 1996 documented excellent tumor-free survival after LT for HCC limited to a single lesion of ≤5 cm or 3 or fewer lesions each ≤3 cm (stage 2 HCC by the TNM system). These so-called Milan criteria were subsequently adopted by the United Network for Organ Sharing, and current LT allocation policy in the United States prioritizes such patients with limited disease. Thus, the patient above with a 2-cm probable HCC might be an ideal candidate for LT.

In patients who do not fulfill the above LT criteria or who are otherwise unsuitable LT candidates, ablation of the HCC can be considered. Some centers also perform ablations of tumors to "buy time" before LT, although this practice remains controversial. Several forms of locoregional ablation have been developed. In the United States, patients with tumors less than (roughly) 6 cm can undergo radiofrequency ablation, either percutaneously or by open laparotomy. The technique delivers energy as heat to the tumor, causing necrosis. Candidate tumors must be relatively peripheral in the liver and not adjacent to major bile ducts or blood vessels. In patients who are deemed at high surgical risk, or in whom the tumor is large (>6 cm) or multiple, transarterial chemoembolization may be considered. The technique takes advantage of the fact that HCCs derive their primary blood supply from the hepatic artery, while the non-tumorous surrounding tissue does not. A catheter is inserted into a branch of the feeding hepatic artery, and chemotherapy is delivered directly into the tumor bed, followed by agents that obstruct the vessel. Many questions remain regarding the effects of locoregional ablation, most importantly whether these procedures, which carry significant risk of morbidity, prolong survival. The indirect and scientifically flawed evidence available, however, suggests that these procedures do favorably affect the survival and management of patients with HCC.

References

1. Borzio M, Fargion S, Borzio F, et al. Impact of large regenerative, low grade and high grade dysplastic nodules in hepatocellular carcinoma development. *J Hepatol.* 2003;39:208-214.
2. Mazzaferro V, Regalia E, Doci R, et al. Liver transplantation for the treatment of small hepatocellular carcinomas in patients with cirrhosis. *N Engl J Med.* 1996;334:693-699.

3. Bruix J, Sherman M, Llovet JM, et al. Clinical management of hepatocellular carcinoma. Conclusions of the Barcelona-2000 EASL conference. European Association for the Study of the Liver. *J Hepatol.* 2001;35:421-430.
4. Bruix J, Sherman M. Management of hepatocellular carcinoma. *Hepatology.* 2005;42:1208-1236.
5. Trevisani F, De NS, Rapaccini G, et al. Semiannual and annual surveillance of cirrhotic patients for hepatocellular carcinoma: effects on cancer stage and patient survival (Italian experience). *Am J Gastroenterol.* 2002;97:734-744.
6. Zhang BH, Yang BH, Tang ZY. Randomized controlled trial of screening for hepatocellular carcinoma. *J Cancer Res Clin Oncol.* 2004;130:417-422.

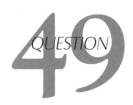

I Have Been Asked to See a Patient Who Had a Liver Transplant 5 Years Ago in Another State. He Has Not Been Seen by His Liver Transplant Center in 2 Years. His Serum Creatinine Is 2.5 mg/dl but His Liver Enzymes and Liver Function Tests are Normal. He Does Not Want to Go Back to His Transplant Center. What Should I Do?

R. Todd Stravitz, MD

Two categories of medical problems must be considered in liver transplant recipients several years after their transplant: allograft-related issues and general medical issues. Five years after orthotopic liver transplant (OLT), allograft-related issues include recurrence of the primary liver disease and less, commonly, chronic rejection or technical complications such as biliary strictures. The single most daunting problem facing liver transplant recipients in 2007 is hepatitis C, the leading cause of cirrhosis and the need for liver transplantation in the United States, which recurs virtually universally after transplant. Compared to the nontransplant population, the natural history of hepatitis C in liver allograft recipients is accelerated, such that up to 30% develop cirrhosis within 5 years of transplant.

Table 49-1

Adverse Metabolic Effects of Common Immunosuppressive Agents in OLT Recipients: Relative Risk*†

Drug	Cyclosporine Neoral, Gengraf	Tacrolimus‡ Prograf‡	Sirolimus Rapamune	MMF CellCept	Cortico-steroids§
Hypertension	+++	+++	−	−	++
Renal Insufficiency	+++	++[1]	−	−	+[2]
Diabetes Mellitus	−	+	−	−	++
Hypercholes-terolemia	+	−	++	−	+
Hypertrigly-ceridemia	+	+/−	+++	−	+
Decreased BMD	++	+	−	−	+++

*BMD indicates bone mineral density; MMF, mycophenolate mofetil.
†Adapted from Sethi A, Stravitz RT. Medical management of the liver transplant recipient: a primer for non-transplant physicians. *Aliment Pharmacol Ther.* 2007;25:229-245.
‡Lower nephrotoxicity of tacrolimus compared to cyclosporine has been reported in several series but remains controversial.
§Corticosteroids may exacerbate calcineurin-induced renal insufficiency by increasing hypertension but do not have direct nephrotoxic effects.

Medical issues facing long-term liver transplant recipients include the development of hypertension, diabetes mellitus, progressive renal insufficiency, decreased bone mineral density, hyperlipidemia, and de novo malignancy. Many of these complications can be ascribed to the immunosuppressive agents administered to all solid organ transplant recipients (Table 49-1). The most prevalent complication of immunosuppressive agents, particularly in patients receiving calcineurin inhibitors (CNIs; cyclosporine A and tacrolimus), is hypertension. By 5 years post-transplant, at least 60% of liver transplant recipients require antihypertensive medications. Chronic renal insufficiency results from several insults to the kidney, including poorly controlled hypertension, new-onset diabetes, and direct toxicity from the CNIs. Early CNI-induced nephrotoxicity results from renal arterial vasoconstriction and is reversible with dose reduction. With time, however, CNI-induced vasoconstriction leads to renal parenchymal ischemia and progressive interstitial fibrosis, which is not reversible. In a large review of solid organ transplant recipients, nearly 20% of liver transplant patients progressed to severe renal failure (glomerular filtration rate of <29 mL/min) within 5 years of their transplant.

The patient presented embodies two commonly coexisting problems in modern liver transplantation: renal insufficiency in the setting of recurrent hepatitis C. The first order of evaluation should be an assessment of modifiable factors that may be contributing to the renal dysfunction. Hypertension, poorly controlled diabetes, and dyslipidemia should be aggressively corrected. Trough serum levels (taken just before the next dose) of CNIs or sirolimus must be assayed, and the transplant center should be contacted with these results so that doses can appropriately adjusted or changes in immunosuppressive regimen discussed. Unless a physician has particular experience with these immunosuppressive agents and their adverse effects, major changes should not be made without the consultation with the transplant center.

Next, specific renal assessment should be undertaken. Consultation with a nephrologist would be reasonable for this patient, especially if urinalysis shows more than slight proteinuria, if dose reduction of the CNI fails to improve serum creatinine, or in the case of difficult-to-control hypertension. CNI-induced renal injury rarely causes significant proteinuria, and its presence suggests a glomerular injury from diabetic nephropathy or other insult. Antihypertensive agents that may be safely used in liver transplant recipients include certain calcium channel blockers (amlodipine or nifedipine preferred), beta-blockers (such as atenolol or metoprolol), and clonidine (Table 49-2). In a transplant recipient with a serum creatinine of 2.5 mg/dL, angiotensin-converting enzyme inhibitors and angiotensin II receptor antagonists should be used cautiously because of the risk of hyperkalemia. At this patient's stage of renal injury, more than one agent may well be necessary to achieve optimal blood pressure control.

After complete medical assessment of the patient presented, the physician should consider assessing the severity of recurrent hepatitis C. If not previously performed, a hepatitis C RNA by reverse-transcriptase polymer chain reaction (RT-PCR) and hepatitis C genotype should be sent to document virologic recurrence of infection. The above patient presents with normal liver-associated chemistries, a reassuring sign that recurrence is relatively mild; progressive hepatic fibrosis from recurrent hepatitis C appears to be more severe in recipients with elevated aminotransferases. However, this observation does not preclude the presence of advanced fibrosis. Therefore, liver biopsy in this patient would be very reasonable.

The presence of fibrosis on liver biopsy should prompt consideration of antiviral therapy, particularly if advanced (bridging fibrosis or cirrhosis). The indications for, and administration of, pegylated interferons and ribavirin in liver transplant recipients remains controversial and should not be undertaken without direct supervision from the liver transplant center or a gastroenterologist with extensive experience with the treatment of hepatitis C and preferably with transplant experience. Antiviral therapy in OLT recipients is often poorly tolerated and risks severe adverse reactions, including precipitation of allograft rejection. Unfortunately, the overall rate of sustained virologic response after antiviral therapy remains disappointingly low.

Table 49-2

Useful Antihypertensive Agents in OLT Recipients: Potential Benefits and Adverse Effects*†

Antihypertensive Aent	*Potential Benefits*	*Potential Adverse Effects*
Calcium-channel blockers	Decreases CNI-induced vaso-constriction	Edema, tachycardia, head-ache, palpitations P450 inter-actions‡
Beta-blockers	Decreases left ventricular hyper-trophy Decreases CNI headache	Impotence, bronchospasm
ACE inhibitors	Renal sparing effect in diabetics Decreases CNI-induced renal fibrosis	Hyperkalemia, azotemia, acidosis
ATII receptor antagonists	Decreases CNI-induced vaso-constriction	Hyperkalemia
Alpha adrenergic agonists (clonidine)	Decreases CNI-induced neuro-genic renal vasoconstriction	Sedation
Thiazide diuretics	Decreases hypervolemia	Hyperlipidemia
Loop diuretics	Decreases hypervolemia	Electrolyte depletion

*CNI indicates calcineurin inhibitors (cyclosporine A and tacrolimus).
†Adapted from Sethi A, Stravitz RT. Medical management of the liver transplant recipient: a primer for non-transplant physicians. *Aliment Pharmacol Ther.* 2007;25:229-245.
‡Cytochrome P450 interactions with CNI result from competition for metabolism and are greatest for diltiazem, verapamil, and nicardipine and least for nifedipine and amlodipine.

References

1. Sethi A, Stravitz RT. Medical management of the liver transplant recipient: a primer for non-transplant physicians. *Aliment Pharmacol Ther.* 2007;25:229-245.
2. Khalid SK, Crippin JS. Management of hepatitis C in the setting of liver transplantation. *Clin Liver Dis.* 2006;10:321-337.
3. Textor SC, Taler SJ, Canzanello VJ, Schwartz L, Augustine JE. Posttransplantation hypertension related to calcineurin inhibitors. *Liver Transpl.* 2000;6:521-530.
4. Ojo AO, Held PJ, Port FK, et al. Chronic renal failure after transplantation of a nonrenal organ. *N Engl J Med.* 2003;349:931-940.
5. Gonwa TA, Mai ML, Melton LB, et al. End-stage renal disease (ESRD) after orthotopic liver transplantation (OLTX) using calcineurin-based immunotherapy: risk of development and treatment. *Transplantation.* 2001;72:1934-1939.
6. Gonwa TA, Mai ML, Klintmalm GB. Chronic renal failure after transplantation of a nonrenal organ. *N Engl J Med.* 2003;349:2563-2565.

INDEX

Printed in the United States
by Baker & Taylor Publisher Services